Copyright © 2016 by Trivium Test Prep

ALL RIGHTS RESERVED. By purchase of this book, you have been licensed one copy for personal use only. No part of this work may be reproduced, redistributed, or used in any form or by any means without prior written permission of the publisher and copyright owner.

Trivium Test Prep is not affiliated with or endorsed by any testing organization and does not own or claim ownership of any trademarks, specifically for the Certified Neuroscience Registered Nurse exam. All test names (and their acronyms) are trademarks of their respective owners. This study guide is for general information and does not claim endorsement by any third party.

Printed in the United States of America

Table of Contents

Introduction 7

Chapter 1: Anatomy & Physiology Review of the Nervous System 9

Chapter 2: Neurological Assessment 21

Chapter 3: Neurological Disorders 25

Chapter 4: Immune and Infectious Disorders of the Neurological System .. 99

Chapter 5: Seizure Disorders 131

Chapter 6: Developmental and Degenerative Disorders 135

Chapter 7: Sleep Disorders 177

Chapter 8: Toxic Encephalopathies 185

Chapter 9: Pain 193

Chapter 10: Chemical Dependency 201

Test Your Knowledge 209

Test Your Knowledge—Answers 233

Exclusive Test Tips 247

Introduction

About the Exam

The Certified Neuroscience Registered Nurse (CNRN) certification provides recognition for a level of excellence in nursing care for neurological patients. CNRNs work with patients throughout all phases of treatment. In order to take the CNRN examination, you need to be a licensed RN who has been employed in neuroscience for two years or for over 4,160 hours. Whether as an administrator or as an educator, you do not need to have any specific continuing education hours for initial certification.

The CNRN test is a computer-based exam offered three times a year (March, July, and October) at approximately 200 sites throughout the U.S. and Canada. To take the exam, members of the American Association of Neuroscience Nurses (AANN) must submit a $250 fee; non-members must submit a $335 fee. The exam contains 220 questions covering all aspects of nursing care for patients with neurological trauma, neurological issues, and rehabilitation.

Once certified, you will hold a valid certification for five years. After that time, you must complete two and a half years of full-time neurological nursing employment and earn 75 continuing-education hours. Additionally, you should recertify with a fee of $215 for AANN members and $300 for non-members.

About Neuroscience Nursing

There are two types of neuroscience nursing practice: direct and indirect. Direct neuroscience is defined as the nursing process in a clinical setting where nursing judgment and actions are more focused on a particular individual or a small group of individuals and where there is a continuing professional responsibility and accountability for the outcomes of various actions. Indirect neuroscience nursing is defined as time spent in clinical supervision of staff or students, consultation, or research.

Patients with insults to the nervous system present with psychosocial, emotional, and physiological needs that require nurses to possess knowledge and competence in order to help them meet the challenges they face in their lives. Neurological nursing is a very challenging nursing specialty dealing with assessment, nursing diagnosis, and management of many neurological disorders for which nurses provide patient care. This includes trauma, brain injuries, stroke, seizures, tumors, headaches, infections, and aneurysms, as well as a host of other neurological complexities (Bader & Littlejohns, 2004).

It is imperative for nurses to have knowledge of neurological disorders and how they influence underlying chronic disease states. Nurses from all specialty settings should stay informed of new and developing treatment modalities, while continuing to review the fundamentals of neurological nursing (Bader & Littlejohns, 2004).

Chapter 1: Anatomy & Physiology Review of the Nervous System

The nervous system is responsible for coordinating all of the body's activities. It controls not only the maintenance of normal functions, but also the body's ability to adapt to external stimuli. The nervous system has three general functions: a sensory function, an interpretative function, and a motor function (Bader & Littlejohns, 2004).

The nervous system is divided into two parts: the central nervous system and the brain. The central nervous system consists of the brain and spinal cord. These structures are protected by bone and cushioned from injury by the cerebrospinal fluid (CSF). The brain is a mass of soft nerve tissue, which is encapsulated within the skull. It is made up of grey matter, mainly nerve cell bodies, and white matter, which are the cell processes. The grey matter is found at the periphery of the brain and in the center of the spinal cord. White matter is found deep within the brain at the periphery of the spinal cord and as the peripheral nerves (Bader & Littlejohns, 2004).

Brain Divisions

- Cerebrum - the largest part of the brain. It is the center for thought and intelligence. It is divided into right and left hemispheres. The right controls movement and activities on the left side of the body. The left controls the right side of the body. Within the cerebrum are areas for speech, hearing, smell, sight, memory, learning, and motor and sensory areas.

- Cerebral cortex - The outside of the cerebrum is called the cerebral cortex. Its function is learning, reasoning, language, and memory.

- Cerebellum - This small structure lies below the cerebrum at the back of the skull. Its functions are to control voluntary muscles, balance, and muscle tone.

- Medulla - The medulla controls heart rate, breathing, swallowing, coughing, and vomiting. Together with the pons and the midbrain, the medulla forms the brainstem that connects the cerebrum to the spinal cord.

- Spinal Cord - The spine is a key part of the nervous system. The spinal cord is a two-foot-long column, which is composed of vertebrae that are separated by intervertebral disks. The spine transverses from the base of the skull and ends with the coccygeal bones (Bader & Littlejohns, 2004).

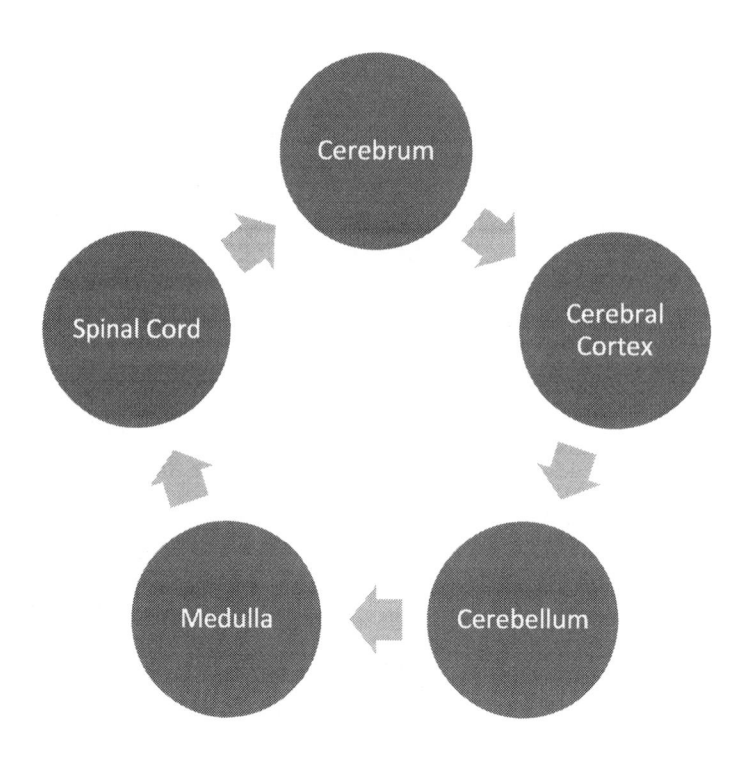

Cerebrum → Cerebral Cortex → Cerebellum → Medulla → Spinal Cord → (Cerebrum)

The Spine

The spine is composed of 33 vertebrae layered with intervertebral disks. The vertebral column creates a hollow tube that encases the spinal cord, making the spinal canal. The layering of the vertebrae creates intervertebral foramina along both sides of the vertebral column, which allows nerves from the spinal cord to exit. The vertebral column is divided into five areas: cervical vertebra 1 through 7 (C1-C7), thoracic or dorsal vertebra 1 through 12 (T1-T12), lumbar vertebra 1 through 5 (L1-L5), sacral vertebra 1 through 5 (S1-S5, fused), and four coccygeal vertebra (fused into one) called the coccyx (Rudyk, McKee, & Lamale, 2013).

All vertebrae are uniform in structure except for C1 and C2. Vertebrae get progressively larger, with the smallest being the cervical vertebrae and the largest being the lumbar vertebrae. The atlas, also referred to as C1, is the first cervical vertebra. This structure supports the head, is ring-like in appearance, has no vertebral body or spinous process, and allows flexion and extension of the head. The axis known as C2 is the second cervical vertebra. This axis has the dens (odontoid process), a small upward projection that connects with C1 to create a pivot and allow the head to rotate. The atlas and axis are connected to each other and the skull by ligaments. Flexion, extension, and rotation are facilitated by the remaining cervical vertebrae, C3 through C7 (Rudyk, McKee, & Lamale, 2013).

The thoracic region of the vertebral column consists of 12 vertebrae (T1-T12). The thoracic vertebrae permit the torso to rotate and bend. Each of the thoracic vertebrae, T1-T10, is connected to a rib. The ribs are not connected to the spine at T11-T12. Due to this lack of attachment, these particular ribs have been nicknamed "floating ribs." The ribs limit the amount of lateral bending by the torso.

The lumbar region of the vertebral column consists of five vertebrae. These vertebrae are large and support the majority of the body's weight. The lumbar vertebrae allow flexion and extension, but they limit rotation of the upper body. The five sacral vertebrae, S1-S5, are fused and form the sacrum. The spine terminates with the remaining five fused vertebrae, which form the coccyx (tailbone) (Rudyk, McKee, & Lamale, 2013).

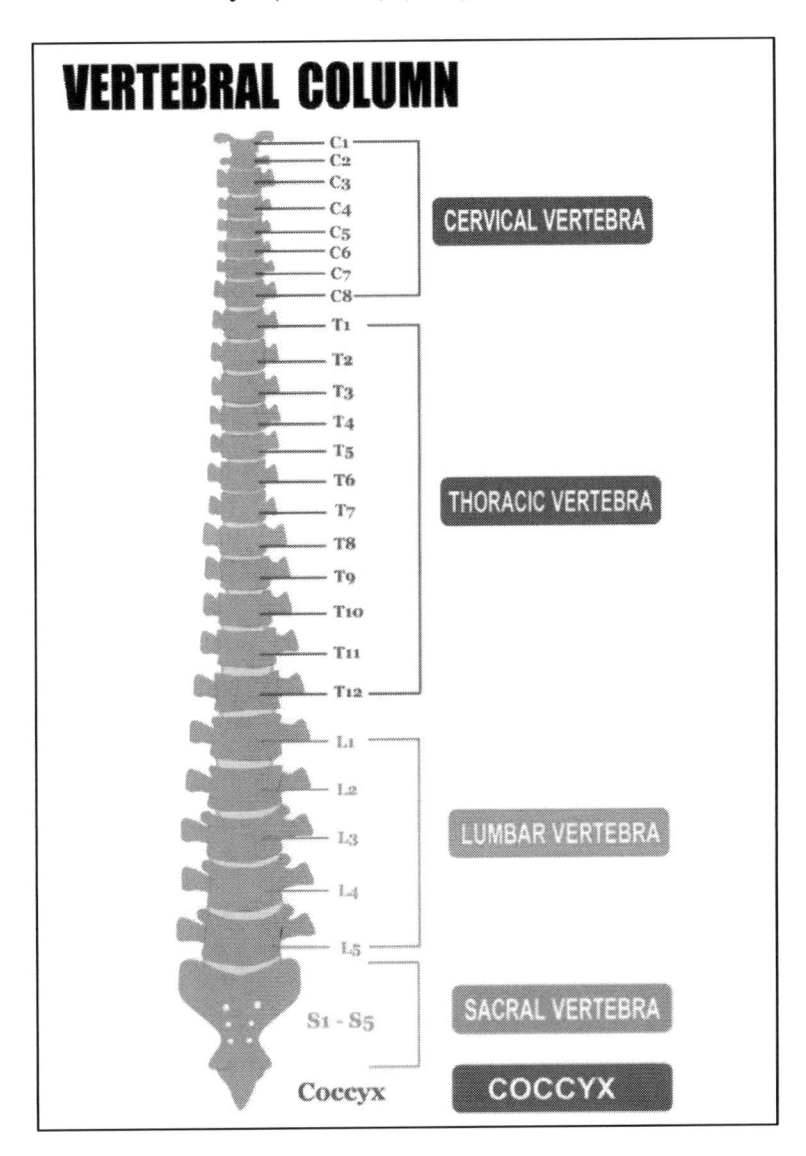

The Peripheral Nervous System

The peripheral nervous system connects the central nervous system to the rest of the body. The main divisions of the peripheral nervous system are the autonomic nervous system, the somatic nervous system, and the nerves.

- The autonomic nervous system - This component controls the automatic functions of the body: the heart, smooth muscle (organs), and glands. It is divided into the "fight-or-flight" system and the "resting and digesting" system.

- The somatic nervous system - This component allows us to consciously or voluntarily control our skeletal muscles. The somatic system contains 12 cranial nerves and 31 spinal nerves.
- Nerves - The nerves are made up of special cells called neurons. Neurons are comprised of a dendrite, a cell body, and an axon. Impulses travel to the dendrite into the cell body and then onto the axon. A special sheath called myelin, which increases the conductivity of the neuron, covers some nerves (Bader & Littlejohns, 2004).

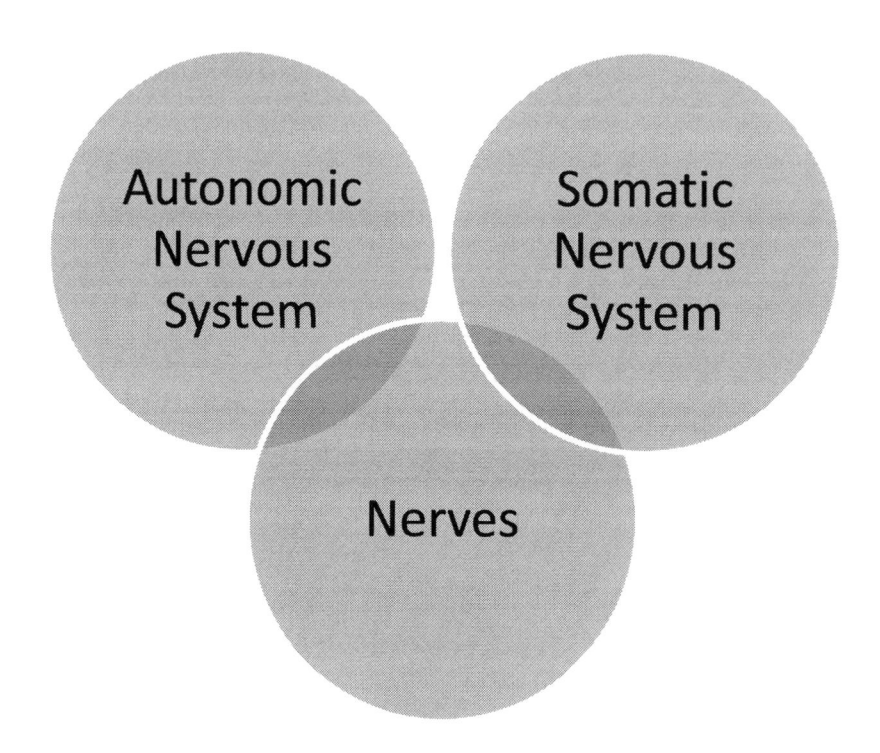

The Parasympathetic Nervous System

- Works to save energy
- Aids in digestion
- Supports restorative, resting body functions
- Decreases heart rate
- Increases gastrointestinal tract tone and peristalsis
- Relaxes urinary sphincter
- Vasodilates vessels
- Decreases blood pressure (Rudyk, McKee, & Lamale, 2013)

The Sympathetic Nervous System

The sympathetic nervous system helps the body cope with external stimuli and functions during stress (triggers the fight or flight response). This system is responsible for:

- Vasoconstriction
- Increasing blood pressure
- Increasing heart rate
- Increasing respiratory rate
- Cold, sweaty palms
- Pupil dilation (Rudyk, McKee, & Lamale, 2013)

The Conduction System

As messages travel from one neuron to the next, they move across a synapse. At each synapse, there is a chemical called a neurotransmitter. At various parts of the body, specific neurotransmitters facilitate communication; for example, dopamine (motor function), serotonin (mood), and endorphins (painkillers). Sensory neurons carry messages from a receptor to the brain. The brain then interprets the message. Motor neurons then send the message to an affector in muscles and glands. During sensory conduction, a receptor (sensory organ) sends a signal to the sensory neuron, which sends a signal to the brain/spinal cord, which then sends a signal to the motor neuron, which sends a signal to the affector (muscle/gland) (Bader & Littlejohns, 2004).

Layers of Defense

- Bones of skull - The neurocranium is comprised of eight bones: occipital, two temporal bones, two parietal bones, sphenoid, ethmoid, and frontal bone. These bones guard the brain.

- Meninges - The meninges are three layers of protective tissue called the dura mater, arachnoid mater, and pia mater that surround the neuraxis. The meninges of the brain and spinal cord are continuous, being linked through the magnum foramen.

- Dura mater - The dura mater is the most superior of the meningeal layers. Its name means "hard mother" in Latin, and it is tough and inflexible. This tissue forms several structures that separate the cranial cavity into compartments and protect the brain from displacement.

- Falx cerebri - This structure separates the hemispheres of the cerebrum.

- Falx cerebelli - This structure separates the lobes of the cerebellum.

- Tentorium cerebelli - This structure separates the cerebrum from the cerebellum (Bader & Littlejohns, 2004).

Sinuses, Dural Spaces, and Mater

The dura mater also forms several vein-like sinuses that carry blood (which has already given its supply of oxygen and nutrients to the brain) back to the heart. The superior sagittal sinus runs across the top of the brain in an anterior-posterior direction. Other sinuses include the straight sinus, the inferior sinus, and the transverse sinus. The epidural space is a potential space between the dura mater and the skull. If there is hemorrhaging in the brain, blood may collect there. Adults are more likely than children to bleed there as a result of closed head injury (Swenson, 2006).

The subdural space is another potential space. It is between the dura mater and the middle layer of the meninges, the arachnoid mater. When bleeding occurs in the cranium, blood may collect there and push down on the lower layers of the meninges. If bleeding continues, brain damage will result from this pressure. Children are especially likely to have bleeding in the subdural space in cases of head injury (Swenson, 2006).

Types of Nervous System Mater

- Arachnoid Mater - The arachnoid or arachnoid mater is the middle layer of the meninges. In some areas, it projects into the sinuses formed by the dura mater. These projections are the arachnoid granulation/arachnoid villi. They transfer cerebrospinal fluid from the ventricles back into the bloodstream.

- Subarachnoid space - The subarachnoid space lies between the arachnoid and pia mater. It is filled with cerebrospinal fluid. All blood vessels entering the brain, as well as cranial nerves, pass through this space. The term arachnoid refers to the spider web-like appearance of the blood vessels within the space.

- Pia Mater - The pia mater is the innermost layer of the meninges. Unlike the other layers, this tissue adheres closely to the brain, running down into the sulci and fissures of the cortex. It fuses with the ependyma, the membranous lining of the ventricles, to form structures called the choroid plexes, which produce cerebrospinal fluid.

- White Mater - White mater is one of the two components of the central nervous system. It consists mostly of glial cells and myelinated axons that transmit signals from one region of the cerebrum to another and between the cerebrum and lower brain centers (Swenson, 2006).

The Limbic System

The limbic system is a convenient way of describing several functionally and anatomically interconnected nuclei and cortical structures that are located in the telencephalon and diencephalon. These nuclei serve several functions; however, most have to do with control of functions necessary for self-preservation and species preservation. They regulate autonomic and endocrine function, particularly in response to emotional stimuli. They set the level of arousal and are involved in motivating and reinforcing behaviors. Additionally, many of these areas are critical to particular types of memory. Some of these regions are closely connected to the olfactory system, since this system is critical to survival for many species (Swenson, 2006).

Frontal Lobe of the Brain

The foremost part of the cortex is the frontal lobe ("prefrontal cortex"), which is responsible for three major functions:

- Executive or higher-level cognitive functioning - This refers to decision-making, planning, organization, and impulse control.

- Working memory - This refers to an attentional system that can hold and manipulate information until it is transferred into long-term storage.

- Personality - This develops over the early years as a function of the interplay between the brain and the environment (Swenson, 2006).

By late adolescence or early adulthood, the personality stabilizes and changes very little over the remaining lifespan. Because of the stability of personality, when individuals do exhibit noticeable changes (e.g. becoming more outgoing, uninhibited, impulsive, socially withdrawn, apathetic), you should be concerned about frontal lobe functioning and refer for further evaluation (Swenson, 2006).

Temporal Lobe of the Brain

The temporal lobe is especially important for:

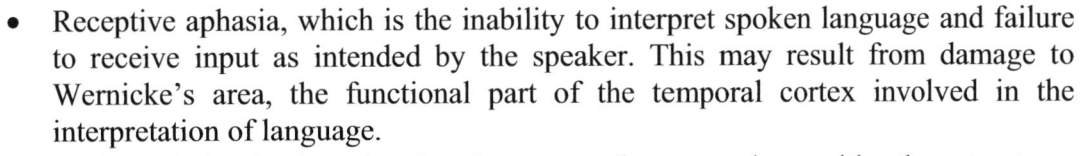

- Hearing, interpreting language, learning and memory, and emotional responses.
- Receptive aphasia, which is the inability to interpret spoken language and failure to receive input as intended by the speaker. This may result from damage to Wernicke's area, the functional part of the temporal cortex involved in the interpretation of language.
- Auditory hallucinations involve the temporal cortex, along with other structures of the brain. Located deep within the temporal cortices are important structures associated with learning and memory (Centers for Disease Control and Prevention, 2013).

Parietal Lobe of the Brain

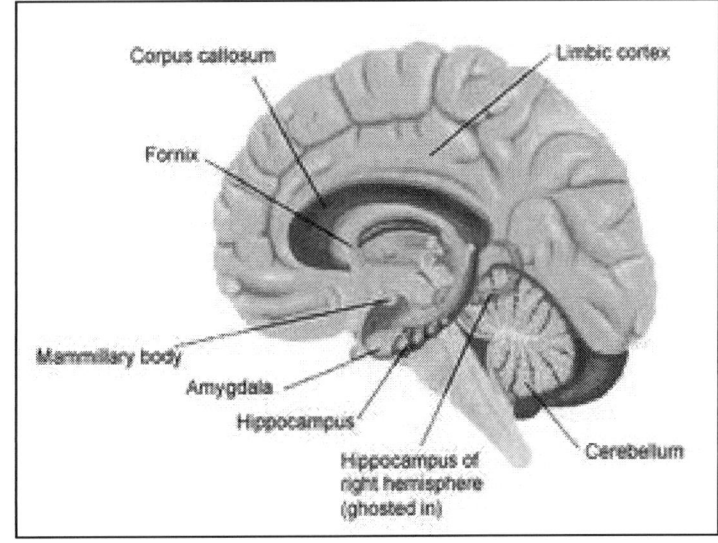

Functions of the parietal lobe include light touch, pressure, pain, temperature, vibration, and proprioception (position sense), which are all somatosensory modalities. The posterior portion of the parietal cortex helps us perceive and interpret spatial relationships, forms an accurate body image (body image disturbances), and learns tasks involving coordination of the body in space. When these areas become damaged, individuals may develop sensory agnosias, defined as the impaired ability to interpret sensory information (identifying a key in one's pocket by touch). Other examples of parietal dysfunction include graphomotor problems (difficulties with drawing a clock or copying a figure) and spatial neglect (often after a cerebrovascular accident) (Swenson, 2006).

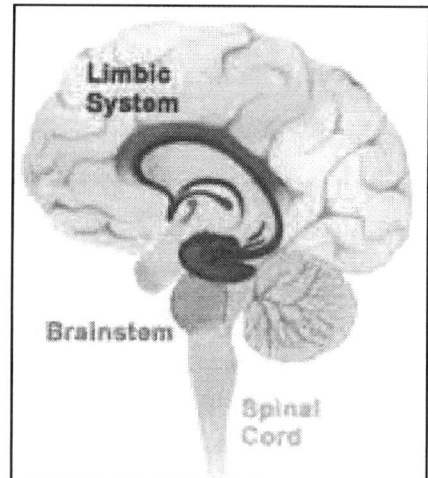

Occipital Lobe of the Brain

Functions of the occipital lobe include visual acuity and visual interpretation from stimulation of the retina. A visual agnosia is the inability to recognize objects through sight. Visual hallucinations involve the visual cortex, along with other brain structures. Damage to this lobe can cause visual problems such as difficulty recognizing objects, identifying colors, and recognizing words (Swenson, 2006).

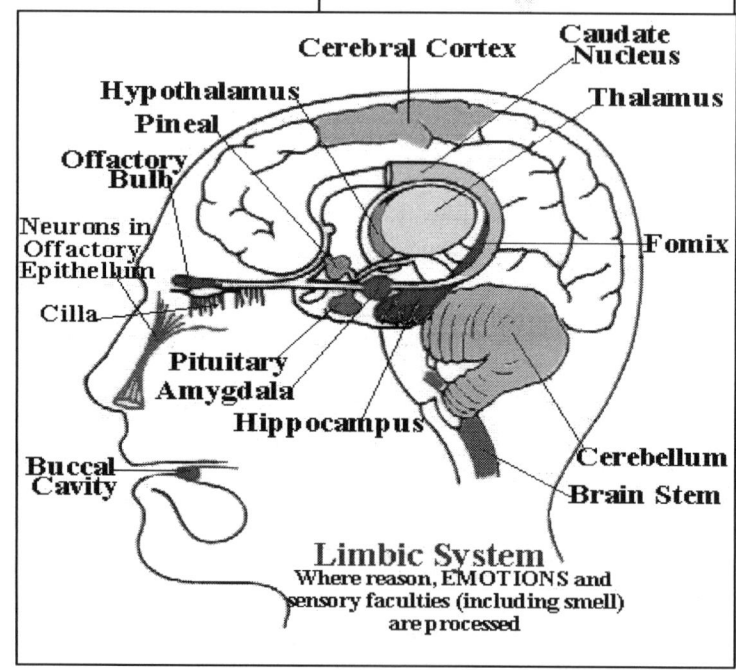

Brainstem

Underneath the limbic system is the brainstem. This structure is responsible for basic vital life functions such as breathing, heartbeat, and blood pressure. The brainstem houses:

- Medulla Oblongata - This structure is the caudal-most part of the brainstem, situated between the pons and spinal cord. It is responsible for maintaining vital body functions such as breathing and heart rate.

- Pons - This is part of the metencephalon in the hindbrain. It is involved in motor control and sensory analysis. For example, information from the ear first enters the brain in the pons. It has parts that are important for level of consciousness and sleep. Some structures within the pons are linked to the cerebellum and thus, are involved in movement and posture.

- Midbrain - This component is involved in functions such as vision, hearing, eye movement, and body movement. The anterior part has the cerebral peduncle, which is a huge bundle of axons traveling from the cerebral cortex through the brainstem. These fibers (along with other structures) are important for voluntary motor function (Centers for Disease Control and Prevention, 2013).

The Reticular Activating System

The reticular activating system (RAS), or extrathalamic control modulatory system, is a set of connected nuclei in the brains of vertebrates that is responsible for regulating arousal and sleep-wake transitions. As its name implies, its most influential component is the reticular formation (Centers for Disease Control and Prevention, 2013).

Cerebellum

The cerebellum is a region of the brain that plays an important role in motor control. It may also be involved in some cognitive functions such as attention and language and in regulating fear and pleasure responses, but its movement-related functions are the most solidly established. The cerebellum does not initiate movement, but it contributes to coordination, precision, and accurate timing. It receives input from sensory systems of the spinal cord and other parts of the brain and integrates these inputs to fine-tune motor activity. Cerebellar damage does not cause paralysis, but instead produces disorders in fine movement, equilibrium, posture, and motor learning (Centers for Disease Control and Prevention, 2013).

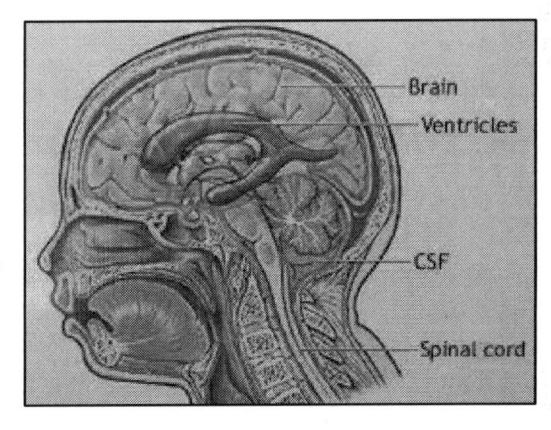

Intracranial Pressure and Cerebral Blood Flow

- CSF - Cerebrospinal fluid (CSF) is a clear liquid produced within spaces in the brain called ventricles. Like saliva, it is a filtrate of blood. It is also found inside the subarachnoid space of the meninges, which surrounds both the brain and the spinal cord. In addition, a space inside the spinal cord called the central canal also contains cerebrospinal fluid. CSF cushions the neuraxis, brings nutrients to the brain and spinal cord, and removes waste from the system.

- Choroid plexus - All of the ventricles contain choroid plexuses, which produce cerebrospinal fluid by allowing certain components of blood to enter the ventricles. The choroid plexuses are formed by the fusion of the pia mater, the most internal layer of the meninges, and the ependyma, the lining of the ventricles.

- Ventricles - These four spaces are filled with cerebrospinal fluid and protect the brain by cushioning it and supporting its weight (Centers for Disease Control and Prevention, 2013).

The Four Ventricles

The two lateral ventricles extend across a large area of the brain. The anterior horns of these structures are located in the frontal lobes. They extend posteriorly into the parietal lobes, and their inferior horns are found in the temporal lobes. The third ventricle lies between the two thalamic bodies. The massa intermedia passes through it, and the hypothalamus forms its floor and part of its lateral walls. The fourth ventricle is located between the cerebellum and the pons (University Hospital, 2013).

- The four ventricles are connected to one another.
- The two foramina of Munro, which are also known as the interventricular foramina, link the lateral ventricles to the third ventricle.
- The Aqeduct of Sylvius, which is also called the cerebral aqueduct, connects the third and fourth ventricles.
- The fourth ventricle is connected to the subarachnoid space via two lateral foramina of Luschka and by one medial foramen of Magendie (University Hospital, 2013).

Subarachnoid Space

Although cerebrospinal fluid is manufactured in all of the ventricles, it circulates through the system in a specific pattern, moving from the lateral ventricle to the third, and then from the third to the fourth. From the fourth ventricle, the cerebrospinal fluid passes into the subarachnoid space where it circulates around the outside of the brain and spinal cord and eventually makes its way to the superior sagittal sinus via the arachnoid granulations, also called arachnoid villi. In the superior sagittal sinus, the cerebrospinal fluid is reabsorbed into the bloodstream. The cerebrospinal fluid of the neuraxis is regenerated several times every 24 hours (University Hospital, 2013).

Endolymph and perilymph, the fluids of the inner ear, are derived from cerebrospinal fluid. Currently, there is no consensus regarding the manner in which cerebrospinal fluid enters the inner ear. Osmosis may be involved, and cerebrospinal fluid can be analyzed to judge a person's general health as can blood and saliva. A sample is taken from the spinal cord via a lumbar puncture, which is also known as a spinal tap (University Hospital, 2013).

Cerebral Circulation

The heart pumps oxygen and nutrient-laden blood to the brain, face, and scalp via two major sets of vessels: the carotid arteries and the vertebral arteries. The jugular and other veins take blood out of the brain. The arteries include:

- The carotid arteries - These vessels run along the front of the neck, one on the left and one on the right. You feel these when you take your pulse just under your jaw. The carotid arteries split into external and internal arteries near the top of the neck.

  - The external carotid arteries - These vessels supply blood to the face and scalp.

  - The internal carotid arteries - These vessels supply blood to the front (anterior) three-fifths of the cerebrum, except for parts of the temporal and occipital lobes.

- The vertebral arteries - These vessels travel along the spinal column and cannot be felt from the outside. They join to form a single basilar artery (hence the name vertebrobasilar arteries) near the brainstem at the base of the skull. These arteries supply blood to the posterior two-fifths of the cerebrum, part of the cerebellum, and the brainstem.

- Other arteries - The arteries that conduct blood to the brain — the internal-carotid and vertebral arteries — connect through the Circle of Willis, which loops around the brainstem at the base of the brain. From this circle, other arteries — the anterior cerebral artery (ACA), the middle cerebral artery (MCA), and the posterior cerebral artery (PCA) — arise and travel to all parts of the brain (University Hospital, 2013).

Because the carotid and vertebrobasilar arteries form a circle, if one of the main arteries is blocked, the smaller arteries that the circle supplies can receive blood from the other arteries. This phenomenon is called collateral circulation, which is a process in which small (normally closed) arteries open up and connect two larger arteries or different parts of the same artery. They can serve as alternate routes of blood supply (University Hospital, 2013).

Sometimes, when an artery in the brain is blocked due to ischemic stroke or transient ischemic attack (TIA), open "collateral" vessels can allow blood to "detour" around the blockage, restoring blood flow to the affected part of the brain. Everyone has collateral vessels, at least in microscopic form. These vessels normally aren't open; however, they grow and enlarge in some people with coronary heart disease or other blood vessel disease. While everyone has collateral vessels, they don't open in all people. The Circle of Willis has a downside, however. Cerebral aneurysms tend to occur at the junctions between the arteries that make up the circle (University Hospital, 2013).

Chapter 2: Neurological Assessment

It is imperative that nurses have a method of assessment to which they can quickly identify problems or changes in their patients. Keen assessment skills help nurses to better communicate with physicians, teammates, and other members of the interdisciplinary team. The purpose of the neurological assessment is to:

- Determine the highest degree of the patient's functional ability and capacity for self-care

- Determine the influence of disability on the patient's and family's lifestyles (Bader & Littlejohns, 2004)

Types of Neurological Assessments

Quick Assessment

- Performed in less than 60 seconds
- Includes PERRLA (pupillary reactivity to light and accommodation), presence of extremity movement, quality of extremity movement, and overall responsiveness (Bader & Littlejohns, 2004)

Limited Assessment

- Screening exam
- Overview of all neurological components, but not detailed
- Includes LOC, hand grips, dorsi/plantar flexion, pupillary size and reaction to light, and eye movements (Bader & Littlejohns, 2004)

Comprehensive Assessment

- Detailed exam
- Includes all neurological components (Bader & Littlejohns, 2004)

Focused Assessment

- Focused on a particular system or anatomic region (coma assessment, brainstem function) (Bader & Littlejohns, 2004)

Assessment Considerations

- Age and developmental level
- Head-to-toe examination
- Environmental influence
- Cultural influences

- Appropriate equipment
- More beneficial observation (Bader & Littlejohns, 2004)

Components of the Neuro Exam

- History
- Source of information (family, witnesses, patient)
- Medical records
- Chief complaint: reason for seeking treatment
- History of present illness
- Temporal development of current complaints
- Onset, duration, frequency, location, and other related symptoms
- Aggravating factors
- Medical/surgical history
- Chronic conditions or diseases
- Past surgical procedures
- History of neurological problems
- Previous injuries
- Familial history of hereditary diseases
- Review of systems
- Inventory of past and present problems of all body systems
- Medications (including OTC and herbal supplements)
- Compliance, response, and adverse effects
- Allergies to medications/substances
- Recreational substances
- ETOH, tobacco, street drugs, and date/time of most recent use (Bader & Littlejohns, 2004)

Physical Assessment

- Level of consciousness (LOC) - A vital component and an early sign of neurological decline.
- Response check - Use verbal or painful stimuli and determine response.
- Glasgow Coma Scale (GCS) - Collective measure of consciousness using eye opening, motor response, and verbal response. GCS score 3 or less indicates coma and is associated with poor outcomes. GCS score 15 means the patient is alert, is awake, and gives an appropriate response.
- Check for understanding - In a normal speaking voice, direct patient to follow commands; you may need to use a louder voice if there is no response.
- Tactile stimulation - This is used if there is no response to auditory stimulation.
- Start with a gentle touch; if there is no response, apply painful stimulation centrally (trap squeeze, pectoralis pressure).
- Deep tactile stimulation - This involves nail bed pressure, sternal rub, or supraorbital notch pressure (may be contraindicated in certain conditions).
- Check orientation - Assess person, place, and time.

Level of Consciousness

- Fully conscious - Awake, alert; oriented to person, time, and place.
- Lethargy - Oriented to place and person, but may be disoriented to time.
- Obtunded - Arouses to stimulation; follows simple commands when stimulated.
- Stupor - Lies quietly with minimal spontaneous movement.
- Unresponsive – Non-mobile except to vigorous stimuli. May respond appropriately to painful stimuli with sounds or eye-opening, but stops responding when stimuli are no longer present.
- Coma - Appears to be in a sleep-like state with eyes closed. Patient does not respond to internal or external stimulation, does not follow commands, has no verbal response or sounds, and his/her motor responses vary depending on severity of coma (Bader & Littlejohns, 2004).

Motor Function

- Localization - Patient follows commands, shows movements away from stimulus, crosses midline, and pushes examiner away.
- Withdrawal - Stimulated limb moves in response to painful stimuli in effort to withdraw from the painful source.
- Abnormal posturing - Patient shows various posturing movements.
- Unresponsiveness - Patient has no signs of reaction to painful stimuli or response (Restrepo, 2008).

Reflexes

Deep tendon reflexes evaluate spinal nerves and include the triceps, biceps, brachioradialis, patellar, and Achilles tendon. Although deep tendon reflexes are not routinely assessed, they should be tested in all patients with a spinal cord injury or with symptoms consistent with a neurological problem (Restrepo, 2008).

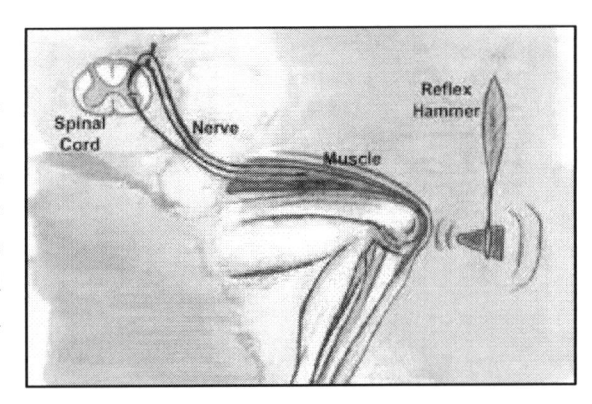

Mental Status/Cognitive Function Assessment

Utilize screening instruments to assess cognitive function and mental status in older adults. These include the Dementia of the Alzheimer Type Inventory, Brief Cognitive Rating Scale, Blessed Dementia Scale, Cognitive Capacity Screening Examination, Cognitive Levels Scale, FROMAJE, Global Deterioration Scale, Mini-Mental State Exam, Clinical Dementia Rating, Mental Status Questionnaire, and Short Portable Mental Status Questionnaire. Also, the neurological nurse should use appropriate, age-specific tools for pediatric and neonatal populations (Bader & Littlejohns, 2004).

Chapter 3: Neurological Disorders

Traumatic Brain Injury

Traumatic brain injury (TBI) is a serious public health disparity in the U.S. Trauma remains the leading cause of death in individuals aged 1 to 44 years, with the majority of injuries being preventable. Annually, traumatic brain injuries contribute to a substantial number of deaths and cases of permanent disability. Every year, at least 1.7 million TBIs occur either as an isolated injury or along with other injuries (Centers for Disease Control and Prevention, 2013; Nayduch, 2009).

A TBI is caused by an impact of force, blow, or jolt to the head or is from a penetrating head injury that disrupts the normal structure and function of the brain. Not all blows or jolts to the head result in a TBI. The severity of a TBI may range from "mild," which generally produces a brief change in mental status or consciousness, to "severe," in which there is an extended period of unconsciousness or amnesia after the injury. The majority of TBIs that occur each year are concussions or other forms of mild TBI (Centers for Disease Control and Prevention, 2013).

Classification of TBI

Severe TBI

- GCS score of 3 to 8
- Motor score < 5 - This occurs when a prolonged unconscious state or coma lasts days, weeks, or months.
- Coma
- Vegetative state
- Persistent vegetative state
- Minimally responsive state
- Akinetic mutism
- Locked-in syndrome (Centers for Disease Control and Prevention, 2013)

Moderate TBI

- Initial severity of injury is prognostic of eventual physical, cognitive, psychosocial, and functional recovery
- Length of stay at least 48 hours
- GCS score of 9 to 12 or higher
- Operative intracranial lesion
- Abnormal computed tomography (CT) scan findings (Bader & Littlejohns, 2004)

Mild TBI

- Also called minor, trivial, or subtle; brain injury is difficult to define

- GCS score greater than 12
- No abnormalities on CT scan
- No operative lesions
- Length of hospital stay less than 48 hours (Bader & Littlejohns, 2004)

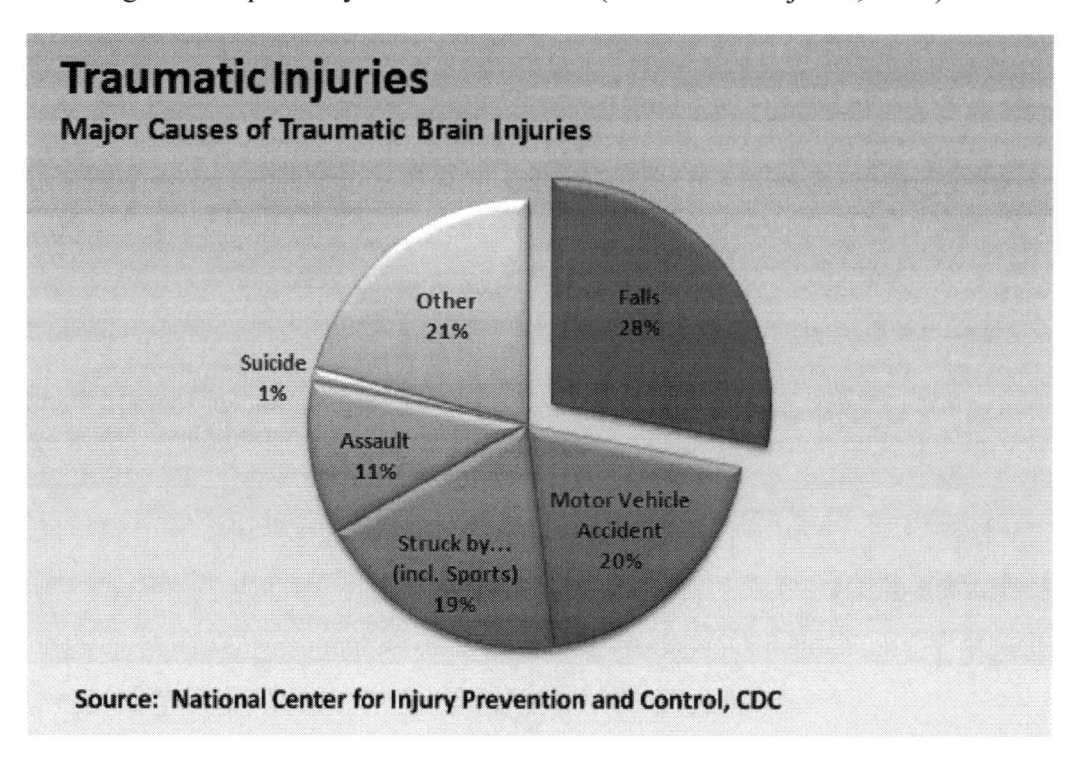

Traumatic Injuries
Major Causes of Traumatic Brain Injuries

- Falls 28%
- Motor Vehicle Accident 20%
- Struck by... (incl. Sports) 19%
- Assault 11%
- Suicide 1%
- Other 21%

Source: National Center for Injury Prevention and Control, CDC

The Leading Causes of TBI

- Falls (28-32%)
- Motor vehicle (17-20%)
- Struck by/against events (16-19%)
- Assaults (11%)
- Suicides (1%) (Centers for Disease Control and Prevention, 2013)

Mechanism of TBI

- Blast - Involves damage to the blood-brain barrier (BBB) and tiny cerebral blood vessels, which are caused by the blood surge moving quickly through large blood vessels to the brain from the torso. Blast damage is a signature war injury in Iraq and Afghanistan. Primary blast injury results from blast wave-induced changes in atmospheric pressure (barotrauma). With a blast injury, organs and tissues of different densities are accelerated at different relative rates, resulting in displacement, stretching, and shearing forces.
- Blunt - Injuries are direct results from an impact with a dull, firm surface or object. The severity of injuries inflicted as a result of blunt force trauma depends on the amount of kinetic energy transferred and the tissue to which the energy is transferred. This may cause contusions and lacerations of the internal organs and

soft tissues, as well as fractures and dislocations of bony structures. Examples of blunt trauma are motor vehicle collisions, falls, and assaults with a blunt object.
- Penetrating - Injuries that result from an object entering the body and sometimes exiting the body, causing damage along the path. The object may not penetrate the fascia, resulting in only an external injury (Batalis & Stephen, 2012; Nayduch, 2009; Weisberg, Garcia, & Strub, 1996).

Severity of TBI

The severity of a TBI may range from "mild," or a brief change in mental status or consciousness, to "severe," or an extended period of unconsciousness or amnesia after the injury (Centers for Disease Control and Prevention, 2013).

The primary injury is defined as the trauma to brain tissue or its vasculature that occurs at the moment of impact. The brain tissue may be injured by direct impact, but most of the damage initiated by the force of primary injury results from sudden motion in the viscoelastic brain. When dynamic forces are involved, injury is more severe. Acceleration/deceleration is abrupt changes in the brain's direction or rate of movement, and direct contact involves injury from a falling object, baseball bat, fist, or the ground (Bader & Littlejohns, 2004).

The extent of injury may be mild with little or no neurological damage or severe with major tissue damage. Unless they are severe, initial forces do not usually cause widespread structural degeneration of neurons, glial cells, or axons. In early post-injury, TBI is largely manifested by brain dysfunction as a result of impaired axoplasmic transport, membrane alteration, and axonal swelling because axonal neuronal destruction is a delayed process (Bader & Littlejohns, 2004).

Types of TBI

- Strain - This follows blunt force, acceleration, deceleration, and rotation of brain tissue. It occurs within the cranial vault, resulting in inertial forces on the brain, shearing of tissues and cellular elements, and production of pressure gradients that are disruptive to brain tissue.
- Variability - This is the nature of the injury produced by strain. It varies according to tissue level and is strain-produced cortical contusions in the gray matter nearest the brain surface.
- Diffuse axonal injury - This takes place in the deeper cerebral white matter where shearing forces cause mechanical and physiological disruption of axons. In the midbrain and brainstem, deep gray matter nuclei and axonal tracts are damaged by strain (Bader & Littlejohns, 2004).

Brain Tissue Compression

- Compressive forces are longer-duration static forces subsequent to brain swelling or hematoma.

- Compression can contribute to alteration in brain function through distortion of tissues, elevation of intracranial pressure, or reduction of perfusion.
- Factors contributing to brain tissue compression include increases in any of the three intracranial components: blood, brain, and cerebral spinal fluid (Bader & Littlejohns, 2004).

Secondary Brain Injury

- Defined as any complicating injury that occurs as a result of further physiological events at some point later in the clinical course.
- Can result from a single neurological event, a series of events, or multisystem complications.
- Involves intracranial (neurological) and extracranial (systemic) processes.
- Many of those with TBI who survive emergency department (ED) arrival will still die within days or weeks as a result of secondary brain injury.
- Severe head injury unleashes a cascade of ischemic and other biochemical changes on the cellular level that can lead to neuronal injury and cell death such as cerebral hypoperfusion, cellular ischemia, hemorrhage, shock states, vasogenic edema, hypermetabolism, infection, hyper/hypocarbia, temperature abnormalities, and inflammation (Centers for Disease Control and Prevention, 2013).

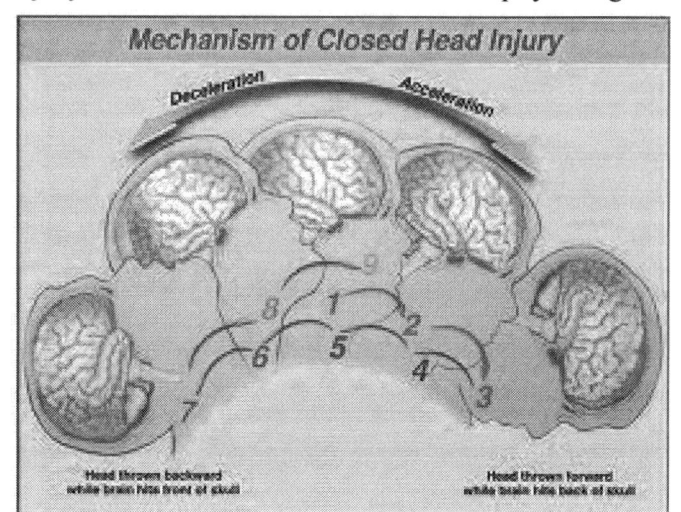

Clinical Presentation – Acute TBI (Mild)

- Appears stunned, dazed, drowsy, or apathetic.
- May be disoriented and have difficulty following complex commands.
- Complains of headache, nausea, vomiting, and/or dizziness.
- Has visual disturbances, amnesia, confusion, tinnitus, irritability, and/or olfactory deficits.
- Has post-concussion syndrome, which appears weeks to months after minor head injury. Symptoms include subtle cognitive and memory difficulties, poor concentration, ease of distraction, slow cognitive processing, susceptibility to internal/external stressors, poor judgment, and/or mental fatigue.
- Can have somatic symptoms such as headaches, dizziness, fatigue, blurred vision, vestibular deficits, nausea and vomiting, neck pain, disorders of smell/taste, and/or hyperesthesias.
- Has affective symptoms such as depression, irritability, decreased drive, anxiety,

emotional labile, impatience, poor frustration tolerance, and/or apathy (Bader & Littlejohns, 2004; Centers for Disease Control and Prevention, 2013).

Clinical Presentation – Acute Moderate-Severe TBI

- Comatose
- Delirious or combative
- Focal neurologic deficits
- Paralysis
- Aphasia
- Visual impairment
- Severe head injury causing severe headache, nausea/vomiting, moaning, groaning, and/or incomprehensible sounds (Bader & Littlejohns, 2004; Centers for Disease Control and Prevention, 2013)

Neurological Assessment and Acute Examination for Severe TBI

- Glasgow Coma Scale
- Eye opening
- Motor response
- Verbal response
- Coma examination
- Observation
- Respiratory patterns
- Spontaneous motor activity
- Seizures
- Posturing
- Eye deviation
- Brainstem function
- CN 2 response to threat
- CN 3, 4, 6, and 8 oculo-cephalic reflex
- CN 5 and 7 corneal reflex
- CN 9 and 10 gag reflex
- Motor/sensory function
- Posturing vs. withdrawal vs. localizing
- Reflexes
- Deep tendon reflexes
- Plantar reflex/babinski
- Signs of psychogenic unresponsiveness
- Forced eye closure
- Nystagmus on caloric testing
- Active resistance to movement
- Avoidance of self-injury
- Catatonia/waxy flexibility (Restrepo, 2008)

Objective Findings

- Pre-hospital information - This includes mechanism of injury, injuries sustained, vital signs, and pre-hospital treatment (MIVT).
- Minor head injury: GCS score of 13 to 15; 30 minutes after the accident, patient is awake and oriented, PERRL, no motor weakness, and no facial deficit
- Moderate head injury: GCS score of 9 to 12
- Severe head injury: GCS score of 3 to 8
- ABCs - Unable to maintain airway
- CO2 retention due to ineffective breathing patterns
- Circulation with increased ICP - Bradycardia, widening pulse pressure, respiratory irregularity due to apnea, tachycardia, hypotension, and apnea
- Decreased LOC, hemiparesis/hemiplegia, flexor or extensor posturing
- Non-reactive pupils, conjugate or disconjugate gaze; facial weakness
- Reflexes - Abnormal with Babinski's reflex

Diagnostic Testing

- Head CT scan
- X-rays - Includes cross-table cervical spine x-ray and chest x-ray
- Diagnostic peritoneal lavage or abdominal ultrasound
- Additional CT scans (abdomen, pelvis)
- Angiography for evaluation of suspected vascular injuries (Bader & Littlejohns, 2004)

Pre-hospital Treatment for TBI

- Rapid stabilization and transport to trauma center
- Complete and rapid physiological resuscitation
- ED management
- Stabilize BP and oxygenation
- Prevent hypotension (keep MAP > 90 mm Hg to maintain presumed CPP > 70 mm HG)
- Prevent/minimize hypoxia (apnea, cyanosis, SpO2 <90% or PaO2 <60 mm Hg)
- Avoid hypotension (MAP <70 mm Hg)
- Hypotension occurring at any time, from initial insult through the acute intensive care course, has been found to be a primary predictor of outcome from severe TBI and is generally the only one that is amenable to therapies. A single hypotension event can DOUBLE mortality and morbidity (Bader & Littlejohns, 2004).

Acute Subdural Hematoma

An acute subdural hematoma (SDH) is a clot of blood that develops between the surface of the brain and the dura mater, the brain's tough outer covering, usually due to stretching and tearing of veins on the brain's surface. These veins rupture when a head injury suddenly jolts or shakes the brain. Traumatic acute SDHs are among the most lethal of all head injuries. Associated with more severe generalized brain injury, they often occur with cerebral contusions. SDHs are seen in 10-20% of all traumatic brain injury cases and occur in up to 30% of fatal injuries. In acute SDHs, which are generally found 48-72 hours after injury, the hematoma is made up of clotted blood and it originates in cortical contusions or tearing of bridging veins or small cortical arteries (Bader & Littlejohns, 2004).

Diagnosis

SDHs are best diagnosed by a CT scan. They appear as a dense, crescent-shaped mass over a portion of the brain's surface. Most patients with acute SDHs have low GCS scores on admission to the hospital. Most of these occur frequently over the frontal, temporal, or parietal convexity (Bader & Littlejohns, 2004).

Treatment

SDHs greater than one centimeter at the thickest point generally require rapid surgical treatment. Smaller SDHs may not require surgery. A large craniotomy, surgery through an opening created in the skull, is often required to remove the thick blood clot and to reach bleeding sites. Cerebral contusions underlying an SDH are often removed during the same surgery (UCLA, 2013).

Outcome

Recovery after brain injury varies widely among patients. The mortality rate for patients with an acute SDH ranges from 50-90%. A significant percentage of these deaths result from the underlying brain injury and pressure on the brain that develops in the days after injury. Approximately 20-30% of patients will recover full or partial brain function. Post-operative seizures are relatively common in these patients. Favorable outcomes are most common in patients who receive rapid treatment, young adults, patients with a GCS score above 6 or 7 and reactive pupils, and those without multiple cerebral contusions or unmanageable pressure on the brain (UCLA, 2013).

Epidural Hematoma

An epidural hematoma (EDH) occurs when blood accumulates between the skull and the dura mater, the thick membrane covering the brain.

Pathophysiology/Etiology

- Usually arterial bleed (middle meningeal artery)
- Typically without parenchymal damage
- Referred to as "talk and die syndrome"
- Typically occur when a skull fracture tears an underlying blood vessel
- EDHs are about half as common as subdural hematomas and usually occur in

- young adults
- Occur four times as often among males than in females and rarely before age 2 or after age 60 (Bader & Littlejohns, 2004)

Symptoms

Classic symptoms of EDH involve brief loss of consciousness followed by a period of awareness that may last several hours before brain function deteriorates, sometimes leaving the patient in a coma. If untreated, the condition can cause increased blood pressure, difficulty breathing, damage to brain function, and death. Other symptoms include headache, vomiting, and seizure (UCLA, 2013).

Diagnosis

Medical personnel typically use CT brain scans to diagnose an EDH, which appears as a dense mass that pushes the brain away from the skull. A magnetic resonance imaging (MRI) scan can also diagnose an EDH, although CT is faster and more commonly used for evaluating trauma patients (UCLA, 2013).

Treatment

A small EDH with no pressure on the brain can be treated without surgery. Severe headache and deterioration of brain function, or an EDH larger than one centimeter at its thickest point, generally indicates surgery is necessary. Surgeons treat EDH by removing the clot to lower pressure on the brain and stopping bleeding to prevent the hematoma from returning (UCLA, 2013).

Diffuse Axonal Injury

Diffuse axonal injury (DAI) is one of the most common and debilitating types of traumatic brain injury. Damage occurs over a more widespread area than in focal brain injury, and extensive lesions in white matter tracts are one of the major causes of unconsciousness and persistent vegetative state after head trauma (Bader & Littlejohns, 2004).

Mechanism of Injury

- Angular acceleration/deceleration
- Stress at gray matter
- Petechial hemorrhages of frontotemporal white matter, corpus callosum, periaqueductal gray, rostral brainstem, putamen, and septum pellucidum
- Axonal shearing and diffuse swelling (Bader & Littlejohns, 2004)

Treatment

There is lack of treatment at this time due to the extent of the diffuse axonal injury.

However, stabilizing the patient and implementing methods to reduce ICP should take priority (Bader & Littlejohns, 2004).

Contusions

Best described as a "brain bruise," contusions can affect only the cortex, or they can involve the subcortical white matter. Most frequently, a contusion occurs in the temporal and frontal regions. However, the most severe occur at the crest of gyri (Bader & Littlejohns, 2004).

Types of Contusions

- Fracture - Most severe, especially in frontal region
- Coup - In point of contact
- Contrecoup - Opposite of contact point
- Herniation - Medical temporal lobe or cerebellar tonsils
- Surface
- Gliding - Focal hemorrhage in cortex and subjacent white matter, found in DAI (Bader & Littlejohns, 2004)

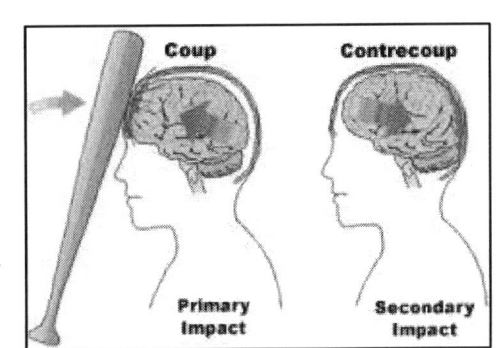

Spinal Column Fractures

Spine fractures can occur from several incidents including falls, osteoporosis, traumatic accidents, spinal tumors, and spinal infections. Many fractures will never require surgery, but major fractures can result in serious long-term problems unless treated promptly and properly (Jacob, Pincus, & Hoh, 2013).

Spine fractures range from painful vertebral compression fractures, often seen after minor trauma in osteoporotic patients, to more severe injuries such as burst fractures and fracture-dislocations, which occur following auto accidents and falls. The basic types of spinal fractures include:

- Vertebral compression fractures
- Vertebral burst fractures
- Fracture-dislocations, which involve significant damage to the facet joints
- Other minor fractures, which consist of laminar, transverse process, or spinous process fractures (Jacob, Pincus, & Hoh, 2013).

Symptoms

Patients complain of significant spinal pain at the level of the fracture. If the fracture compresses the spinal cord or spinal nerve roots, there can be pain, numbness, reflex changes, and weakness in the distribution of skin and muscle supplied by that nerve. A significant traumatic spinal fracture may cause a spinal cord injury, resulting in paralysis

(Jacob, Pincus & Hoh, 2013).

Diagnosis

Performing a detailed neurological examination can determine if the spinal cord or spinal nerves are compressed. Spinal fractures are easily diagnosed by plain x-rays of the spine as well as CT scans of the spine. MRI is often used to look for associated disc herniation or bleeding (Jacob, Pincus & Hoh, 2013).

Treatment

Many fractures heal with conservative treatment. Severe fractures may require surgery to realign the spine. The decision to treat a spinal fracture is based on whether there are any neurological symptoms, such as weakness, and whether the spine is unstable. If the bone fragments are pressing on the spinal cord or nerve roots, prompt surgery is indicated. Severe fractures may involve several columns of support in the spine, which will require surgical fixation to regain stability (Jacob, Pincus & Hoh, 2013).

Surgical fixation involves both instrumentation and fusion, which is the joining of two vertebrae with a bone graft (either from the patient or from cadaver) held together with metal hardware such as plates, rods, hooks, screws, and cages.

The goal of the bone graft is to join the vertebrae above and below to form one solid piece of bone; this may take several months or longer to create a solid fusion. The instrumentation holds the bones together while the fusion is taking place. Smoking cessation is highly encouraged to aid in successful fusion (Jacob, Pincus & Hoh, 2013).

If there is no neurological deficit or instability, surgery may be deferred and simple external bracing will suffice. Braces maintain spinal alignment, immobilize the spine during healing, and control pain by restricting movement.

Stable fractures may require only stabilization with a brace such as a rigid neck collar (Aspen collar) for cervical fractures, a cervical-thoracic brace (Minerva brace) for upper back fractures, or a thoracolumbar-sacral orthosis (TLSO) for lower back fractures. After 8-12 weeks, the brace is usually discontinued (Jacob, Pincus & Hoh, 2013).

Progressive deformity or pain is an indication for surgery. This minimally invasive procedure is called a kyphoplasty, which re-expands the vertebral body and augments its strength by injecting bone cement. In other cases, cement injection without re-expansion of the fracture, called vertebroplasty, can be performed (Jacob, Pincus & Hoh, 2013).

Nursing Interventions

- Assess for history of the injury, presence of factors that may cause pathologic fractures (osteoporosis, osteomyelitis, neoplastic diseases, etc.)
- Look for presence of signs of fracture (edema, pain, loss of motion, crepitus,

extremity disproportion, or abnormal positioning)
- Assess presence of signs and symptoms of soft tissue involvement (swelling, hemorrhage, impaired sensation in the extremity)
- Assess extremity for presence of open fracture and severe external hemorrhage
- Assess vital signs, fluid balance, and urine output
- Assess diagnostic tests and procedures for abnormal values
- Assess routine preoperative history
- Provide emergency care if required (hemostasis, respiratory care, prevention of shock)
- Provide fracture fixation to prevent following injury of tissues
- Observe signs of fat embolism (especially during first 48 hours after the fracture)
- Monitor fluid input and output continuously by inserting IV catheter and urinary catheter
- Monitor client vital signs
- Monitor client laboratory test results for abnormal values
- Administer IV therapy, analgesics, antibiotics, and other medications as prescribed
- Prepare client and family for surgical intervention if required
- For client after surgical intervention, provide routine post-operative care and teach about possible post-operative complications
- Provide care to client with cast (observe signs of circulatory impairment such as changes in skin color and temperature, diminished distal pulses, pain, and swelling of the extremity and protect the cast from damage)
- Provide care to client in traction (check that weights are hanging freely, observe skin for irritation and site of skeletal traction insertion for signs of infection, and use aseptic technique when cleaning the site of insertion)
- In case of hip fracture and hip replacement, maintain adduction of the affected extremity
- Provide respiratory exercises to prevent lung complications
- Observe for signs of thrombophlebitis and report immediately
- Provide appropriate skin care to prevent pressure sores
- Encourage fluid intake and high-protein, high-vitamin, high-calcium diet
- Teach proper techniques for braces and external devices
- Teach client appropriate crutch-walking techniques
- Provide emotional support to patient and family
- Explain all procedures to decrease anxiety and to obtain cooperation
- Instruct client regarding fracture healing process, diagnostic procedures, treatment and its complications, home care, daily activities, diet, restrictions, and follow-up (Bader & Littlejohns, 2004)

Skull Fractures

- Skull fracture - Any break in the cranial bone as a result of trauma.
- Linear fracture - Associated with milder brain injury and is relatively common in infancy.

- Depressed fracture - Displaced greater than half the width of the bone and is often associated with contusions underlying the fracture.
- Basilar fracture - Occurs in the base skull (frontal, ethmoid, sphenoid bone). Patient gets raccoon eyes or panda eyes, which is called periorbital ecchymosis (Bader & Littlejohns, 2004).

Complications of Skull Fractures

- Rhinorrhea - CSF leak and blood
- Otorrhea - CSF and blood
- Hemotympanum
- Conductive hearing loss
- "Battle sign" - Ecchymosis over mastoid process
- Peripheral nerve palsy - Due to injury to cranial nerve VII (Bader & Littlejohns, 2004)

Spinal Cord Injury

Spinal cord injury (SCI) occurs as a result from compression, tearing, ischemia, or laceration of the spinal cord, resulting in permanent or temporary loss of normal sensory, motor, or autonomic function. Spinal cord edema may further compromise neurological function (Bader & Littlejohns, 2004).

Factors that affect Morbidity and Mortality

- Age at onset of SCI
- Level of injury
- Neurological grade (based on number of muscles affected, degree of motor weakness, and presence of sensory impairment)
- Patients with higher lesions with neurological deficits have higher mortality rates.
- Elderly patients have higher mortality rates (Bader & Littlejohns, 2004).

Epidemiology - Incidence

- 11,000 SCIs occur each year in the U.S.
- Half of SCI patients are 16-30 years old
- Median age is 26 years
- Mean age is 31.7 years
- Males are more likely than females to sustain SCI
- Non-traumatic (malignancy and AV malformations) SCI is more likely to occur in patients older than 40 years of age

Epidemiology - Prevalence

- In the U.S., 190,000 live with SCIs
- Average life expectancy:

- High tetraplegics live, on average, 33 years after injury
- Low tetraplegics live, on average, 39 years after injury
- Paraplegics live, on average, 44 years after injury
- Elderly patients (>60 years) with SCI live, on average, 7-13 years after injury, depending on the level of injury (Bader & Littlejohns, 2004)

Etiology and Causative Factors

- Motor vehicle crashes (MVCs) - 44%
- Interpersonal violence - 24%
- Falls - 22%
- Sports-related incidents - 8%
- Diving tends to be associated with cervical SCI
- Parachuting tends to be associated with thoracolumbar SCI
- Other causes - 2% (industrial incidents, crush injuries) (Bader & Littlejohns, 2004)

Mechanisms of Injury

- Hyperflexion injuries are often associated with sudden deceleration (head-on MVC, diving incident).
- Rotational injuries caused by extreme flexion rotation or lateral flexion of the spine disrupt the posterior ligaments, producing spinal instability.
- Hyperextension injuries typically result from falls or rear impact MVCs.
- Axial loading/vertical compression occurs when overwhelming vertical force is applied to the vertebral body, causing burst fractures.
- Penetrating injury violates the spinal column and may allow direct cord contact.
- Stab wounds, gunshot wounds, and shrapnel (Bader & Littlejohns, 2004).

Associated Damage with SCI

Soft tissue injury can be classified as:

- Ligamentous - Can cause spinal cord instability
- Muscular - Paraspinal muscle spasm may provide temporary stability to the spinal column

Vertebral Injuries

- Simple fracture - Single break in the spinal process.
- Compression fractures - Cause flattening or wedging of the vertebral body, but are generally stable.

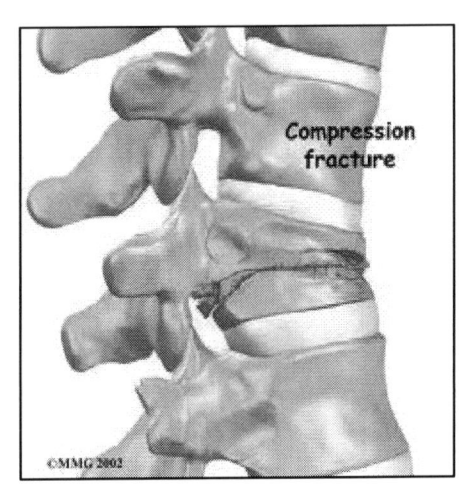

37

- Teardrop fractures - Small chip of bone off the anterior inferior edge of the vertebral body and are unstable.
- Atlas fractures
- Jefferson fractures - C1 burst fractures, which may be managed with external orthotic device.
- Axis fractures
- Odontoid fractures - Occur after extreme flexion, rotation, or extension; rarely associated with SCI.
- Hangman's fracture - Involve fractures through the bilateral pedicles of C2 resulting from hyperextension of the neck; neurological impairment is rare.
- Fracture dislocations - Caused by hyperextension or hyperflexion with or without rotation.
- Rotary subluxation - Caused by abnormal rotation at the C1-C2 complex; the patient may exhibit torticollis, which may be difficult to see on plain film (Bader & Littlejohns, 2004).

Classification of SCI

- Concussion - Transient loss of spinal cord function.
- Contusion - Involves intramedullary hemorrhage and associated edema.
- Laceration - A cut of the spinal cord.
- Transection - A complete cut through the cord; very rare.
- Hemorrhage - May occur into the parenchyma of the spinal cord or one of the meningeal layers.
- Vascular damage to vessels, which perfuse the spinal cord. This can result in spinal cord ischemia (Bader & Littlejohns, 2004).

Classification of SCI by Functional Loss

- Complete injuries - Result in the loss of all voluntary motor and sensory function below the level of injury.
- Incomplete injuries - Allow some neurotransmission distal to the level of injury and can be classified based on the type of function preserved.
- Central cord syndrome - Usually results from hyperextension injuries to the cervical spine, which causes injury and edema in the center of the spinal cord.
- Motor loss - Is greater in the upper extremities than in the lower, and bladder dysfunction and variable sensory loss are also present. Also, recovery is variable, with worse outcomes if patient is > 50 years old, is 70 years of age or older, or has a poor prognosis at discharge.
- Anterior spinal artery syndrome - Is associated with disruption of the arterial supply to the anterior two-thirds of the spinal cord, resulting in infarction to this portion of the cord. Symptoms include paralysis, loss of touch, pain, and temperature sensations below the injury. Light touch sensation may be present as well as proprioception and preservation of vibration.
- Brown-Sequard syndrome - Is related to hemisection of the spinal cord resulting from penetrating injury. It may result from ischemia, infection, or hemorrhage and

has a variable recovery. Symptoms include loss of motor function (i.e. hemiparaplegia), loss of vibration sense and fine touch, loss of proprioception (position sense), loss of two-point discrimination, and signs of weakness on the ipsilateral (same side) of the spinal injury.
- Dorsal column syndrome - Involves damage to the posterior aspect of the spinal cord.
- Horner's syndrome
- Conus medullaris syndrome
- Cauda equina syndrome (Bader & Littlejohns, 2004)

Pathophysiology

Primary injury occurs from biomechanical forces of trauma that destroy neurons and their support cells. Injury can cause immediate hemorrhage and cell death, which causes ischemia. Secondary injury occurs from physical destruction and ischemia caused by primary injury, which triggers a cascade of secondary processes that exacerbate damage over hours to weeks after initial insult. Other contributing factors include:

- Electrolyte shifts
- Excitatory amino acids
- Inflammatory processes
- Spinal shock
- Acute spinal cord injury
- Absence of all voluntary and reflex neurologic activity below level of injury
- Decreased reflexes
- Loss of sensation
- Flaccid paralysis below injury
- Lasts days to months (transient)
- Spinal shock and neurogenic shock in the same patient
- Neurogenic shock
- Hemodynamic phenomenon - Loss of vasomotor tone and loss of sympathetic nervous system tone
- Impaired cellular metabolism (Bader & Littlejohns, 2004)

Critical Features

- Hypotension - Due to massive vasodilation.
- Bradycardia - Due to unopposed parasympathetic stimulation.
- Poikilothermia - Unable to regulate temperature, which occurs within 30 minutes after cord injury at the level T5 or above, and lasts up to 6 weeks; it is also due to some drugs that affect vasomotor center of medulla such as opioids or benzodiazepines (Bader & Littlejohns, 2004).

Management

- Determine underlying cause

- Airway support
- Fluids as needed - Typically 0.9 NS, where the rate depends on need
- Atropine for bradycardia
- Vasopressors such as phenylelphrine (neo-synephrine) for BP support (Bader & Littlejohns, 2004)

Spinal Cord Assessment

- Initial assessment of airway patency, ventilation, and circulation.
- Gross neurological assessment (during initial resuscitation phase).
- Once stable, perform full neurological assessment.
- Initial full neurological assessment serves as a baseline for future evaluations.
- Deterioration in neurological function is common.
- Early deterioration is often related to treatment (traction, inadequate immobilization).
- Delayed deterioration (24 hours to 7 days) is associated with hypotension in patients with fracture locations.
- Late (>7 days) deterioration may be associated with vertebral artery injuries.
- Changes in examination warrant further investigation.
- Assess sharp vs. dull in each dermatome and proprioception (position sense) (Bader & Littlejohns, 2004).

ASIA International Standards

- Sacral sparing
- Reflexes
- Cutaneous reflexes
- Priapism
- Vital sign alterations
- Bradycardia
- Hypotension
- Reduced respiratory effort
- Temperature abnormalities (Bader & Littlejohns, 2004)

Diagnostics

- X-ray films obtained for initial evaluation of the spinal axis (AP & lateral views)
- CT
- MRI
- Myelogram - Invasive test that involves the injections of water-soluble contrast media into the subarachnoid space under fluoroscopy. This assesses for nerve root lesions, nerve root avulsions, the subarachnoid space, intravertebral disc herniation, vertebral dislocation, and spinal cord compression.
- Studies to assess vasculature such as angiography (Bader & Littlejohns, 2004)

Medical Interventions

- Initial immobilization used during resuscitation
- Firm backboard
- C-collar
- Specific stabilization devices
- Hard cervical collars
- Cervical traction
- Halo vest
- Cervicothoracic orthoses
- Thoracolumbosacral orthoses (Bader & Littlejohns, 2004)

Surgical Intervention

- Can be safely performed in the first 24 hours
- Vertebrectomy - burst injuries
- Diskectomy and fusion for decompression of traumatic disk herniation
- Laminoplasty to decompress the cord
- Fusion to provide stability if the posterior ligaments have been disrupted (Bader & Littlejohns, 2004)

Medications

- Solumedrol (methylprednisolone)
- GM-1 ganglioside
- Vasopressors to normalize blood pressure
- Technology to improve function and fitness
- Tendon transfers
- Functional electrical stimulation (FES)
- DVT prophylaxis (Bader & Littlejohns, 2004)

Multidisciplinary Team Approach Treatment

- RN, physician specialists, RT, ST, PT, OT, and case management
- Respiratory support
- Secretion control
- Mechanically assisted cough
- External neuromuscular stimulation
- Suctioning
- Chest physiotherapy
- Bronchoscopy
- Ventilator support
- Noninvasive support with oxygenation and ventilation in patients with respiratory muscle fatigue
- Invasive support with positive pressure mechanical ventilation
- C5 "keep the diaphragm alive" - Any injury above C5 will require mechanical

- ventilation during acute phase
- Chronic ventilator support - 5% of all new SCI will require lifelong support
- Positioning and mobilization
- Kinetic therapy
- Supine position (especially during spinal shock)
- Sitting position
- Abdominal binders (increase tidal volume, inspiratory capacity, total lung capacity)
- Incentive spirometry
- Resistive inspiratory muscle training (Bader & Littlejohns, 2004)

Nursing Interventions

- Promote adequate breathing and airway clearance.
- Monitor pulse oximetry and ABGs.
- Clear bronchial and pharyngeal secretions.
- Use suctioning cautiously, which can stimulate the vagus nerve, causing bradycardia.
- Chest physiotherapy and breathing exercises
- Humidification
- Adequate hydration
- Assess for signs of respiratory infection.
- Intubate and ventilate (Bader & Littlejohns, 2004)

Improve Mobility

- Maintain proper alignment at all times.
- Reposition frequently.
- Prevent foot drop by having the patient wear shoes.
- Prevent external rotation of hip joints with trochanter rolls.
- Prevent contractures by performing range of motion exercises 4 times daily.
- If injury is above midthoracic level, monitor BP when turning (loss of sympathetic control of peripheral vasoconstriction) (Bader & Littlejohns, 2004).

Maintain Urinary and Bowel Function

- Intermittent or indwelling catheter to avoid over-distention of bladder
- Urinary retention results from bladder becoming atonic.
- Intake and output
- Insert NG tube to relieve distention and prevent aspiration.
- Paralytic ileus usually develops.
- Bowel activity usually returns within one week.
- High-fiber, high-protein diet
- Stool softener (Bader & Littlejohns, 2004)

Managing Potential Complications

Thrombophlebitis and Pulmonary Embolism
- Assess for symptoms (chest pain, dyspnea, ABGs)
- Measure circumference of thighs and calves daily
- Anticoagulation (low dose heparin)
- Pressure stockings
- Adequate hydration

Orthostatic Hypotension
- BP unstable and low for first two weeks must be monitored
- Have patient wear pressure stockings (Bader & Littlejohns, 2004)

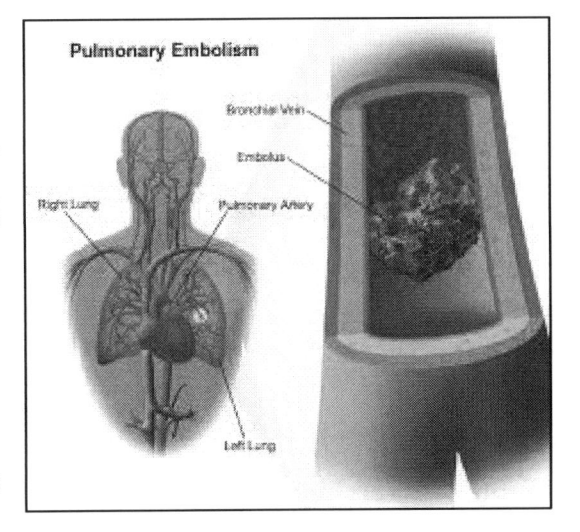

Autonomic Hyperreflexia

- Exaggerated autonomic response
- Causes severe headache, hypertension, profuse diaphoresis, nausea, nasal congestion, and bradycardia
- Can be triggered by distended bladder, distended bowel, and stimulation of skin
- Immediate action required by placing patient in sitting position
- Alleviate cause (empty bladder, check rectum, examine skin for areas of pressure and irritation)
- Treated with apresoline (ganglionic blocking agent) (Bader & Littlejohns, 2004)

Herniated Nucleus Pulposus

A herniated nucleus pulposus (HNP), also referred to as a herniated disc, is a common spine pathology that occurs approximately 95% of the time at the L4-L5 or L5-S1 level. The peak incidence of HNP is 30-55 years of age. The majority of herniated discs occur in a posterolateral direction, compressing the ipsilateral nerve root as it exits the dural sac. A tear in the outer, fibrous ring (annulus fibrosus) of an intervertebral disc (discus intervertebralis) allows the soft, central portion (nucleus pulposus) to bulge out beyond the damaged outer rings. This is usually due to age-related degeneration of the annulus fibrosus, although trauma, lifting injuries, and straining have been implicated (Bader & Littlejohns, 2004).

Radiculopathy

Radiculopathy is pain, paresthesias, or both in the distribution of a nerve root. Patients typically describe deep buttock, posterior, or posterolateral thigh pain that may or may not extend below the knee into the lower leg and lateral foot. The pain is often aggravated by coughing, sneezing, or straining. It may also be aggravated by certain positions such as sitting or standing. The pain usually subsides with rest (Bader & Littlejohns, 2004).

Cauda Equina Syndrome

Symptoms of cauda equina syndrome include urinary retention or incontinence; saddle anesthesia; progressive leg or foot weakness–often bilateral; and bowel incontinence, which is rare. Neurologic compromise from this syndrome is severe and represents a surgical emergency (Bader & Littlejohns, 2004).

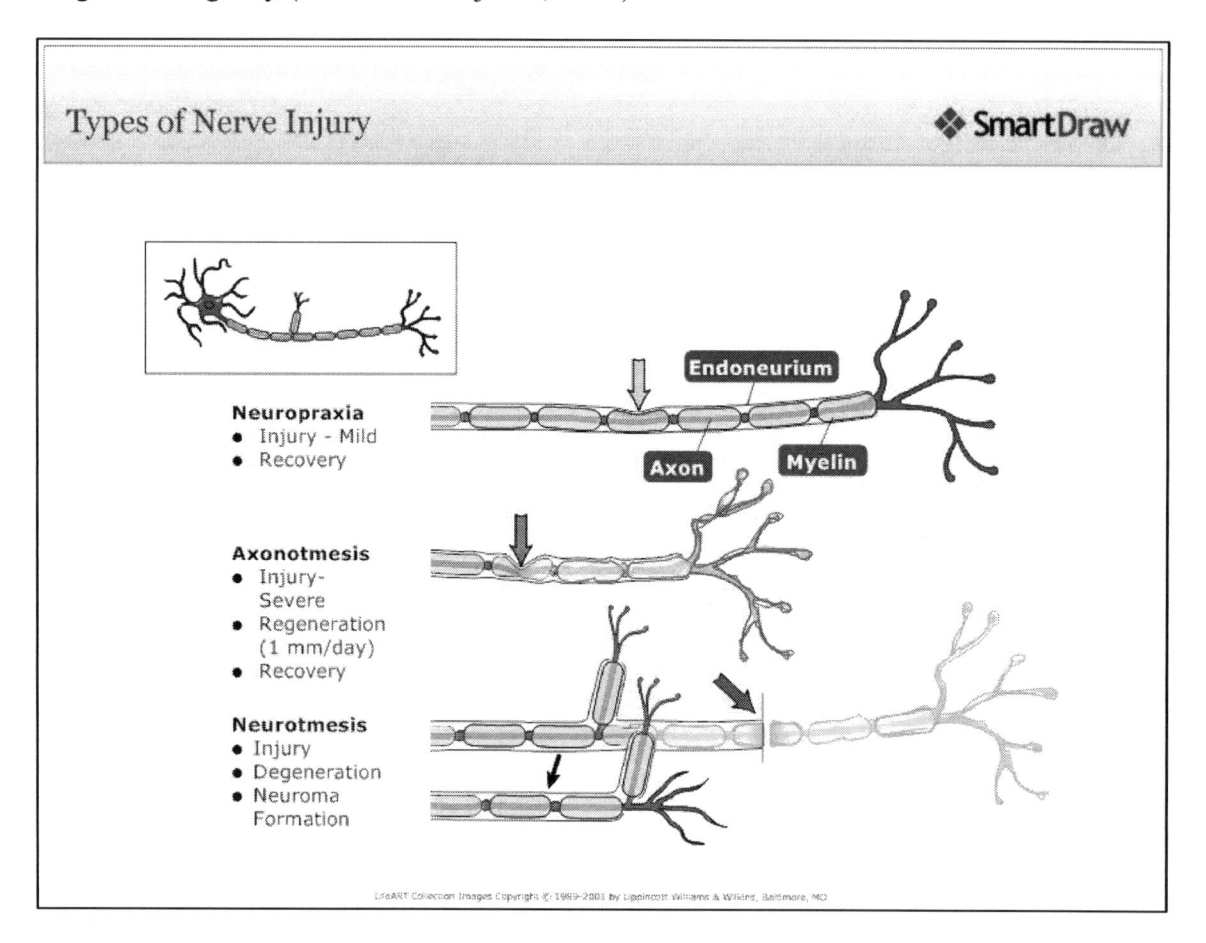

Types of Nerve Injury

- Neuropraxia
  - Injury - Mild
  - Recovery
- Axonotmesis
  - Injury- Severe
  - Regeneration (1 mm/day)
  - Recovery
- Neurotmesis
  - Injury
  - Degeneration
  - Neuroma Formation

Peripheral Nerve Injury

Peripheral nerve injury can occur through a variety of trauma. Common causes of nerve injuries include:

- Laceration
- Focal contusion (gunshot wounds)
- Stretch/traction injury
- Compression
- Drug injection injury
- Electrical injury (John Hopkins University, 2013)

Types of injury

- Brachial Plexus injury - Is injury to the brachial plexus nerve.

- Foot drop injury - Is injury to the peroneal nerve and sciatic nerve.
- Meralgia paresthetica - Is injury to the lateral femoral cutaneous nerve and femoral nerve.
- Spinal accessory nerve injury - Is injury to the spinal accessory nerve and cranial nerve.
- Traumatic nerve injury (John Hopkins University, 2013)

Diagnosis of a Nerve Injury with the Sunderland Classification System

The Sunderland Classification System divides nerve injuries into five parts:

- First-degree injury: A reversible local conduction block at the site of the injury. This injury does not require surgical intervention and usually will recover within a matter of hours up to a few weeks.
- Second-degree injury: There is a loss of continuity of the axons or electrical wires within the nerve. If this kind of injury can be confirmed through preoperative nerve testing, surgical intervention is usually not required.
- Third-degree injury: There is damage to the axons and their supporting structures within the nerve. In this case, recovery is variable. Intraoperative nerve conduction studies are often able to help predict outcome and need for simple cleaning of the nerve (neurolysis) or a more extensive repair with grafting.
- Fourth-degree injury: In this case, there is damage to the axons and the surrounding tissues sufficient to create scarring that prevents nerve regeneration. Intraoperative electrical testing confirms that no electrical energy can be passed along the neural pathways in this injured nerve. Surgical intervention with nerve grafting is necessary to repair the damage.
- Fifth-degree injury: These injuries are usually found in laceration or severe stretch injuries. The nerve is divided in two. The only way to repair a fifth-degree injury is through surgery (John Hopkins University, 2013).

Diagnostic Testing

In order to fully determine the extent of the damage to the nerve, an EMG/NCV (an electrical conduction test) may be used to determine the passage of electrical currents through the nerves. These tests are sometimes completed during actual surgery while the patient is sedated. Other tests include CT, MRI, and neurography (John Hopkins University, 2013).

Treatment for Nerve Injuries

- Acupuncture
- Massage therapy
- Medication
- Orthotics
- Physical therapy and rehabilitation
- Weight loss management (John Hopkins University, 2013)

Surgery for Nerve Injuries

The goal of surgical repair is to repair the nerves so that function is restored to the area. Surgery is often delayed in cases of blunt lacerations so that nerve action potential studies can be used to document the absence of regeneration. Surgery is performed early in cases of sharp lacerations and involves nerve grafting with delayed cases. Grafting after six months is associated with poorer outcomes (Bader & Littlejohns, 2004).

Repetitive Stress Injury - Carpal Tunnel Syndrome

With carpal tunnel syndrome (CTS), the median nerve is compressed by swelling of irritated/inflamed tendons and other structures (venous engorgement) in the rigid carpal tunnel. Acute CTS presents with severe pain, wrist or hand swelling, cold hand, and decreased finger motion. Chronic CTS is the most common, and it presents with motor and sensory dysfunction atrophy (flattening of the muscle at the ball of the thumb) (Bader & Littlejohns, 2004).

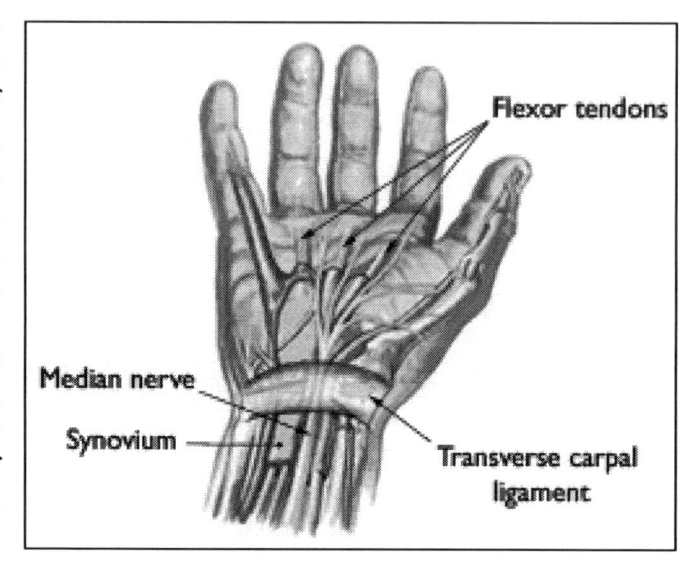

Epidemiology of CTS

- Most common in peripheral nerve entrapment syndrome
- Prevalence varies by occupation, industry, and state
- Peaks between 30 and 50 years of age (Bader & Littlejohns, 2004)

CTS Etiology and Contributing Factors

- Associated with highly repetitive work, forceful work, and exposure to vibration
- Younger - Repetitive stress injury
- Older - Idiopathic
- Rarely familial
- Predisposing factors
- Autoimmune/hematological
- Multiple myeloma
- Sarcoidosis
- Blood dyscrasias
- Rheumatoid disease
- Congenital anomalies

- Idiopathic
- Infectious/inflammatory
- Tuberculosis
- Tenosynovitis
- Metabolic/hormonal
- Pregnancy
- Diabetes mellitus
- Acute renal failure
- Dialysis
- Neoplasms
- Trauma
- Vascular (Bader & Littlejohns, 2004)

CTS Prevention

- Frequent rest periods when using repetitive movements
- Proper body and limb alignment
- Proper use of padding during surgical procedures or instances where limbs may be in a fixed position for an extended amount of time
- Principles of ergonomics used in office space design (Bader & Littlejohns, 2004)

Assessment for CTS

- Entrapment injuries
- Determine mechanism of injury
- Acute symptoms include burning, lancing, tearing, and piercing pain
- Chronic symptoms include dull, throbbing, and aching pain, which may last for years
- Determine functional limitations
- Prior treatments, therapies, and medication history (Bader & Littlejohns, 2004)

Examination for CTS

- Test strength and motor function
- Test sensation
- Tinel's sign - Tapping the regenerating axons of the injured nerves elicits a tingling or paresthesia distal to the injured nerve.
- Impaired function
- Absence of sweating
- Skin changes
- Observe for muscular atrophy (Bader & Littlejohns, 2004)

Anatomy of the Carpal Tunnel:

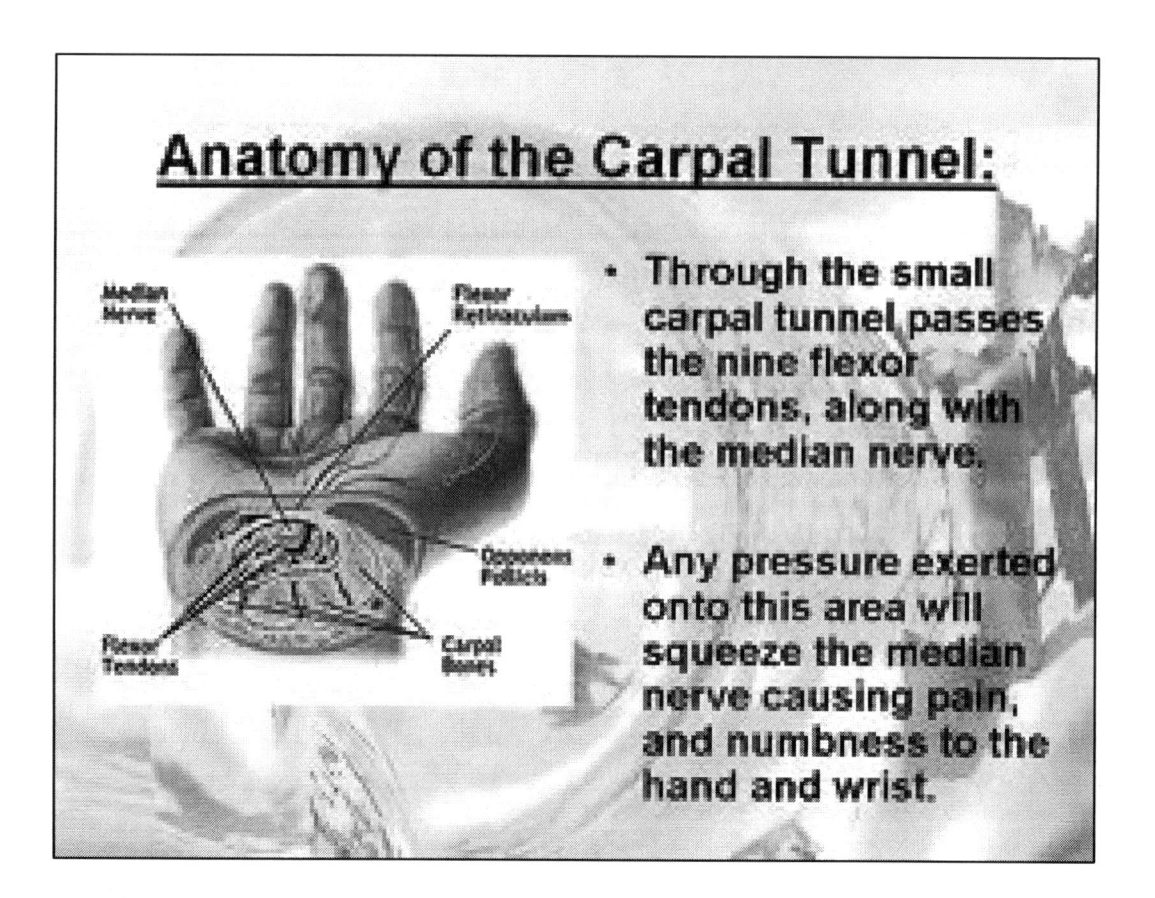

- Through the small carpal tunnel passes the nine flexor tendons, along with the median nerve.
- Any pressure exerted onto this area will squeeze the median nerve causing pain, and numbness to the hand and wrist.

Diagnostics for CTS

- Electrophysiological testing
- NCS/EMG (Bader & Littlejohns, 2004)

Medical and Nursing Interventions

- Immobilization with splint
- NSAIDs
- Diuretics if limb swelling is a problem
- Ergonomic redesign
- Steroid and/or lidocaine injections if no response to conservative measures; may be repeated in 7-10 days
- Skin care for surgical patient
- Provide pain management
- Assess neurovascular status
- Teach about splinting (Bader & Littlejohns, 2004)

Stroke

Is my patient having a TIA? A stroke? What are my next steps? Review how to perform stroke assessment and the ABCs of managing these life-threatening attacks.

The management and treatment of cerebrovascular disease is a rapidly progressing science. The advancement of technology, strategies, and treatment modalities are surfacing more quickly than they can be learned by healthcare providers such as neurological nurses. Modern literature reveals that the longer the delay between the onset of symptoms and the initiation of treatment, the higher the probability of complications, morbidity, and mortality related to cerebrovascular insults. Strokes are typically classified as either vessel rupture (hemorrhagic) or vessel occlusion (ischemic) (Bader & Littlejohns, 2004).

Impact of Stroke

In the U.S., there are nearly 700,000 cases of stroke per year, making the event the third leading cause of death among the population. Over half of these cases are first-time insults, and approximately a quarter of these cases are recurrent attacks. Currently, a "brain attack" occurs every 45 seconds, and every 3.1 minutes, someone dies as a result of a stroke. The average cost of stroke-related medical expenses and disability is approximately $51 billion. Strokes are the leading cause of serious, long-term disability in the U.S, and nearly half of all hospitalized patients are admitted for acute neurological events (Bader & Littlejohns, 2004).

Stroke Prevention

In order to reduce stroke-related health disparities, a strategically coordinated effort among healthcare providers in communities has emerged. Such efforts include integrated emergency response systems, public education, and multidisciplinary treatment modalities. Nurses play a vital role in prevention by communicating assessment findings and educating the at-risk population. Healthcare systems can further focus efforts by implementing cultural awareness of stroke prevention by providing ongoing continuing-education for clinical staff. Emphasis on the recognition of non-modifiable risk factors (age, sex, race, ethnicity, and family history) can also promote prevention (Bader & Littlejohns, 2004).

Patients should be counseled on the following modifiable risk factors:

- Hypertension (HTN) should be treated aggressively to maintain SBP below 140 mm Hg and DBP below 90 mm Hg.
- Diabetes mellitus control
- Smoking cessation
- Coronary artery disease, cardiac arrhythmias, CHF, and valvular disease should be treated.
- Reduction of alcohol use/abuse
- Use of oral contraceptives should be discontinued or, at minimum, changed for a low-estrogen dose.
- Post-menopausal estrogen replacement should not be discontinued.
- Hyperlipidemia should be treated in order to reduce coronary artery disease.
- Physical inactivity must be corrected, and the benefits of exercise should be

discussed (Bader & Littlejohns, 2004).

Stroke Assessment

Neurological assessment of the patient with stroke-like symptoms is critical to prevent the potential injury of brain tissue or to preserve tissue that remains viable. Nurses cannot rely on technology or monitors to adequately assess patients during neurological events. A systematic approach to assessing patients with neurological disorders should include:

- Subjective data - The patient may not report any symptoms listed previously, so careful attention to medical history is critical because diagnosis is generally based on clinical history alone.
- Objective data - There is often no objective data by the time the patient is seen by a healthcare provider.
- Diagnostic data - Used for patients > 50 years of age without an obvious diagnosis on initial exam (Bader & Littlejohns, 2004).

Diagnostic Evaluations

The recommended initial diagnostic evaluations are:

- CBC with platelet count
- Chemistry profile (including fasting cholesterol level and glucose tolerance)
- Prothrombin time (PT)
- Activate partial thromboplastin time (PTT)
- Erythrocyte sedimentation rate (ESR)
- Syphilis serology
- Electrocardiogram (ECG)
- CT scan (particularly in hemispheric TIAs)
- Noninvasive arterial imaging (ultrasound)
- Magnetic resonance angiography (MRA) (Bader & Littlejohns, 2004)

Common Contributing Factors

- Unrecognized seizures
- Confusional states
- Syncope
- Hypoglycemia
- Drug overdose
- Hyponatremia
- Hypoglycemia
- Migraine
- Concussion with head injury
- Encephalopathies or encephalitis
- Eclampsia

- Brain tumors
- Subdural hematoma
- Determine NIH stroke scale (Bader & Littlejohns, 2004)

Transient Ischemic Attack

Transient ischemic attack (TIA) is defined as a neurological deficit lasting <24 hours that is related to focal cerebral or retinal ischemia. Nearly 90% of TIAs resolve within 10 minutes of onset. During a TIA, there is ischemia to the brain from various causes outlined in etiology. Signs and symptoms correlate with the region of the affected cerebral blood flow. The hallmark is that there is no permanent deficit or damage, thus making it "transient." Major causes of TIAs are atrial fibrillation, carotid artery disease, large artery disease, small artery disease, hypercoagulable states, and drug use (Bader & Littlejohns, 2004).

TIA Classifications

Anterior circulation symptoms:

- Carotid artery - Contralateral motor and sensory loss and/or transient blindness (amaurosis fugax) or transmonocular blindness caused by emboli to retinal artery.
- Anterior cerebral artery (ACA) - Confusion, personality change, incontinence, and contralateral motor or sensory loss in leg greater than arm.
- Middle cerebral artery (MCA) - Contralateral motor or sensory loss (arm greater than leg), contralateral motor loss in lower face, contralateral visual field loss, language loss (dominant hemisphere), and spatial-perceptual loss (non-dominant hemisphere).
- Posterior cerebral artery (PCA) - Contralateral motor or sensory loss, ipsilateral visual field loss, cortical or bilateral blindness, dysarthria, dysphagia, diplopia, and quadreparesis.
- Vertebrobasilar circulation - Symptoms correlate with brainstem and cerebellar functions including cranial nerve deficits for CN III-XII, ataxia, bilateral blindness or hemianopsia, confusion, diplopia, bilateral limb weakness, bilateral paresthesias, slurred speech, and vertigo (Bader & Littlejohns, 2004).

Patient Problems

1) Risk for altered cerebral tissue perfusion - nearly 30% of patients with TIAs will have a stroke within five years
    - Goal is to prevent future stroke (Bader & Littlejohns, 2004).

Interventions
Medications:
- Antiplatelet agents: Aspirin 50-325 mg daily, Plavix 75 mg daily, Aggrenox 25 mg twice daily

- o Anticoagulants: Warfarin sodium (Coumadin) with goal INR of 2.5 for Atrial fibrillation
- o tPA for thrombotic strokes (three-hour window from onset of symptoms)

Surgical Interventions:
- o Carotid Endarterectomy
  - o The *most* beneficial for symptomatic patients with severe carotid stenosis (70-99%)
  - o Beneficial for symptomatic patients with moderate carotid stenosis (50-69%)

Nursing Interventions
- o Start O2, IV; cardiac enzymes also
- o Evaluate three-hour window or IV tPA

Acute Care
- o Assess and monitor neurological status for any further signs and symptoms of altered cerebral tissue perfusion
- o Facilitate and educate patient and family about diagnostic procedures

Expected Outcome
- o Patient has a reduced risk of recurrent TIA and future stroke (Bader & Littlejohns, 2004).

2) Knowledge deficit related to recommended lifestyle modifications, new medication regimen, or surgical procedures
   - o The patient who experienced a TIA needs appropriate information to make lifestyle changes designed to prevent recurrent TIAs and future stroke

Interventions
Medical Therapy
- o Prescription for and explanation of antiplatelet or anticoagulant agent

Surgical Therapy
- o Recommendation for and explanation of carotid endarterectomy

Nursing Interventions
- o Assess patient and family for baseline knowledge level of recommended medications and procedures
- o Educate patient and family according to assessment of knowledge deficit; health literacy appropriation
- o Provide educational materials based on literacy level
- o Educate patient about risk factors; emphasis: blood pressure control, diabetes self-care, limiting alcohol intake, treating heart disease, monitoring cholesterol, exercise, nutrition, and stopping use of illicit drugs

Expected Outcome
- o The patient and family are knowledgeable about recommended medications, procedures, and risk factors; the patient and family can verbalize the warning signs of a stroke (Bader & Littlejohns, 2004).

Aneurysm

An aneurysm is known as an abnormal dilatation of a blood vessel that is at risk of enlargement and rupture. Saccular, or berry, aneurysms are most common types of cerebral aneurysms (Bader & Littlejohns, 2004).

Classification

- Location
    - o 85% anterior circulation - ACA (anterior communicating artery), posterior communicating artery, MCA, and their branches
    - o 15% posterior circulation - vertebral artery, basilar artery, posterior cerebral artery, and their branches; these usually occur at arterial bifurcations
- Shape
    - o Saccular, or berry, aneurysm: well-defined neck; arises from one artery; 80-90% of all aneurysms; narrow or wide neck
    - o Giant aneurysm: ≥25 mm; may involve more than one artery; may attach to multiple perforating branches
    - o Fusiform aneurysm: involves the normal wall of an artery; no defined neck; most common in vertebrobasilar system
    - o Dissecting aneurysm: elongated dilatation of an artery that involves injury to normal layers of artery wall; generally related to trauma
    - o Mycotic aneurysm: infectious aneurysm; rare; septic emboli from bacterial endocarditis (Bader & Littlejohns, 2004)

Epidemiology

- Prevalence among population is 0.5-5% in U.S. (Bader & Littlejohns, 2004)

Pathophysiology

- Hemodynamics and growth
    - o Aneurysm formation is influenced by various hemodynamic factors (shear stress, pressure, and impingement force)
    - o Also influenced by humoral factors (inflammatory mediators and adhesion molecules)

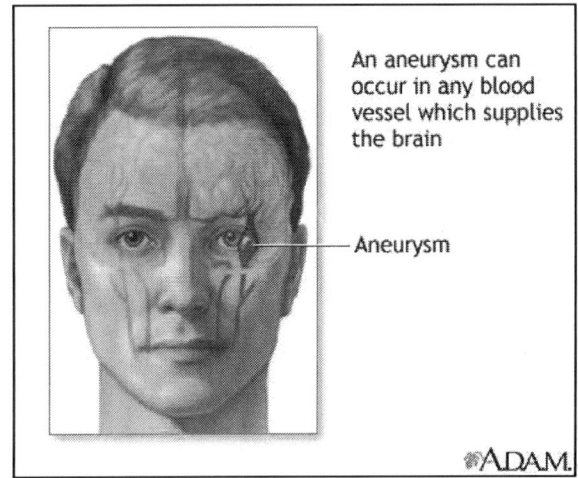

- Aneurysm growth is not well understood and is affected by the integrity of the arterial wall and hemodynamic force (Bader & Littlejohns, 2004)

Assessment

- Subjective
  - Symptomatic:
    - CN deficits include oculomotor paresis secondary to mass effect from large or giant cavernous sinus aneurysms; ptosis: mass effect on adjacent CN III posterior communicating artery aneurysm
    - Transient ischemic events from embolus from large or giant aneurysms
  - Asymptomatic: Truly incidental (two thirds of asymptomatic aneurysms)
    - Usually are evaluated first for dizziness, headache, motor vehicle accidents
    - Evaluation because of familial history of ASAH
- Objective
  - History: personal history, familial history, genetic problems, tobacco use, headaches rarely associated with incidental aneurysms
  - Physical assessment: comprehensive neurological assessment; usually non-focal, may have CN deficits as mentioned earlier
- Diagnostic
  - Noninvasive screening: MRI brain, MRA brain
  - Invasive: CTA; four-vessel cerebral angiogram is the gold standard (Bader & Littlejohns, 2004)

Interventions

- Surgical
  - Preferred therapy for most aneurysms; 98% cure rate
  - Hospital stay is three to five days
- Medical
  - Surgeon to address risk and benefit with patient and family
  - Post-operative analgesia
  - Evaluation of post-operative CT scan
  - Follow up with serial MR angiograms at one-year or two-year intervals
  - Maintenance of BP within designated range (SBP 110-150 mm Hg)
- Nursing
  - Critical care: monitor neurological status at least hourly; administer pain medications as prescribed; monitor and document the response; position for comfort every two hours and as circumstances require; provide non-pharmacological remedies as needed (ice packs)
  - Acute care: continue observance of neurological status; continue use of pain scale assessments; advance diet; manage pain; begin discharge teaching to patient and family members
  - Rehabilitation is not applicable on elective clipping unless there are complications (Bader & Littlejohns, 2004)

- Endovascular therapy/coiling
    - Rapidly evolving technology
    - 70-80% cure rate
    - Less post-operative discomfort
    - Carries same risks of morbidity and mortality as a craniotomy (Bader & Littlejohns, 2004)

Arteriovenous Malformation

- Arteriovenous malformation - cerebral
- A cerebral arteriovenous malformation is an abnormal connection between the arteries and veins in the brain that usually forms before birth (Bader & Littlejohns, 2004)

Etiology

- The cause of cerebral arteriovenous malformation (AVM) is unknown. The condition occurs when arteries in the brain connect directly to nearby veins without having the normal vessels (capillaries) between them.
- Arteriovenous malformations vary in size and location in the brain.
- An AVM rupture occurs because of pressure and damage to blood vessel tissue. This allows blood to leak into the brain and surrounding tissue and reduces blood flow to the brain.
- Cerebral AVMs occur in less than 1% of people. Although the condition is present at birth, symptoms may occur at any age. Hemorrhages occur most often in people ages 15-20, but can also occur later in life. Some patients with AVMs also have cerebral aneurysms (Bader & Littlejohns, 2004).

Symptoms

In about half of patients with AVMs, the first symptoms are those of a stroke caused by bleeding into the brain.

Symptoms of an AVM that is not bleeding are:

- Confusion
- Ear noise/buzzing (also called pulsatile tinnitus)
- Headache in one or more parts of the head; may seem like a migraine
- Problems with walking
- Seizures
- Symptoms due to pressure on one area of the brain
- Blurred, decreased, or double vision
- Dizziness
- Muscle weakness in any part of the body or face
- Numbness in any part of the body

- o Exams and tests
  - A complete physical examination and neurological examination are needed, but may be completely normal (Bader & Littlejohns, 2004)

Diagnostics

- o Cerebral angiogram
- o CT angiogram
- o Cranial MRI
- o Electroencephalogram (EEG)
- o Head CT scan
- o MRA
- o Magnetic resonance veinogram (Bader & Littlejohns, 2004)

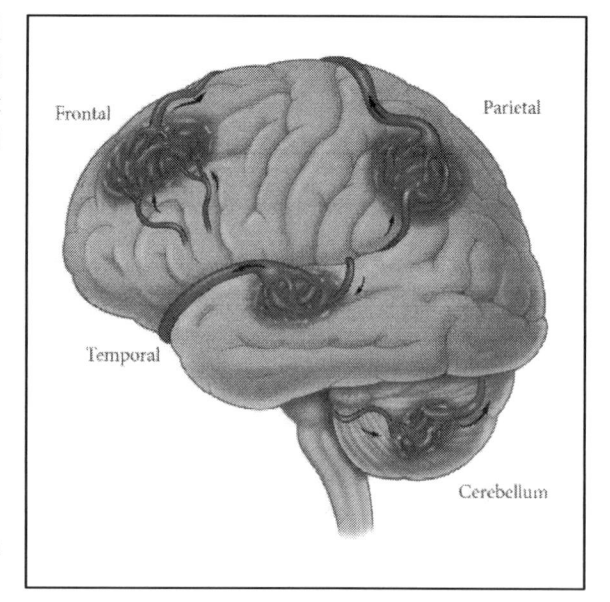

Treatment

- A bleeding AVM is a medical emergency. The goal of treatment is to prevent further complications by controlling bleeding and seizures and, if possible, removing the AVM.
- Three surgical treatments are available. Some treatments are used together.
  - o Open brain surgery - Removes the abnormal connection through an opening made in the skull. It must be done by a highly skilled surgeon.
  - o Embolization (endovascular treatment):
    - A catheter is guided through a small cut in your groin to an artery and then to the small blood vessels in your brain where the aneurysm is located.
    - A glue-like substance is injected into the abnormal vessels to stop blood flow in the AVM and reduce the risk of bleeding. This may be the first choice for some kinds of AVMs or if surgery cannot be done.
  - o Stereotactic radiosurgery:
    - This procedure delivers very focused radiation directly to the area of the AVM to cause scarring and shrinkage.
    - It is particularly useful for small AVMs deep in the brain, which are difficult to remove by surgery.
    - Anticonvulsant medications, such as phenytoin, are usually prescribed if seizures occur (Bader & Littlejohns, 2004).

Arteriovenous Fistula

- An arteriovenous fistula, or DAVF, is an abnormal connection of vessels in the tissues around the brain or spinal cord in which one or more arteries are directly connected to one or more veins or venous spaces called sinuses (John Hopkins University, 2013).

Dural Arterialvenous Fistula

- A form of spinal AVM and dura
- Occurs in the dural root sleeve
- Comprises 80-85% of all spinal AVMs
- Male predominance; occur between ages 40 and 60
- Present as a radiculomyelopathy with progressive neurological deterioration
- A single or multiple dural artery feed vessel contributes to high venous outflow pressure, resulting in venous dilation and spinal ischemia
- Treatment is surgical - Dura is opened, fistula is coagulated and removed; preoperative embolization (Bader & Littlejohns, 2004)

Etiology

- In a DAVF, there is a direct connection between one or more arteries and veins or sinuses, which causes many problems.
- Arteries carry blood from the heart to the tissues, and veins take blood back from the tissues to the heart.
- DAVFs differ from AVMs; AVMs are found within the tissue of the brain or spinal cord, and DAVFs are found in the coverings of the brain or spinal cord such as the dura mater or arachnoid.
- The most serious problem associated with DAVFs is that they transfer high-pressure arterial blood into the veins or venous sinuses that drain blood from the brain and spinal cord.
- This results in increased pressure of the venous system around the brain and spinal cord (John Hopkins University, 2013).

Symptoms

- There are two major types of AVFs: dural AVFs and carotid-cavernous fistulas (CCFs).
- These are acquired lesions, which are lesions that patients are not born with, but instead develop later in life.
- They can be a result of infection or traumatic injuries, but most develop without any specific precipitating event.
- Patients with dural AVFs typically present with a rumbling noise in one ear that follows the heartbeat, which is called a bruit.
- Patients with CCFs typically present with swelling and redness of one or both eyes in addition to a bruit (John Hopkins University, 2013).

Diagnosis of Arteriovenous Fistula (DAVF)

- Whenever possible, the main attempt is to close the DAVFs before the increased pressure in the venous system causes irreversible damage to the brain or spinal cord.

- Obtain an angiogram. An angiogram (also called an arteriogram) is a special test in which a neuroradiologist injects dye into the blood vessels in the brain to obtain images of the blood vessels.
- Currently, the angiogram is the test that most accurately shows the DAVF and its relationship to the surrounding arteries and veins. In the case of most DAVFs, the CT and MRI scans are often read as normal (John Hopkins University, 2013).

Treatment of Arteriovenous Fistula

- Minimally invasive endovascular embolization — typically sufficient to cure the majority of DAVFs.
- During this procedure, a catheter is passed through the groin up into the arteries in the brain that lead to the DAVF and injects liquid embolic agents such as NBCA, glue, or Onyx into these arteries. This injection shuts off that artery and reduces the flow of blood through the DAVF.
- Microsurgical resection — reserved for DAVFs that cannot be closed with endovascular embolization. During microsurgical resection, a craniotomy is performed and, using a microscope, the DAVF is isolated from the tissues around the brain and spinal cord (John Hopkins University, 2013).

Carotid Stenosis

Carotid artery stenosis is a common diagnosis in general medical practice (Lanzino, Rabinstein, & Brown, 2009).

Symptoms

In daily clinical practice, carotid artery stenosis is found in many patients during evaluation of ill-defined episodes of "dizziness," generalized subjective weakness, syncope or near-syncope episodes, "blurry vision," or transient positive visual phenomena (such as "floaters" or "stars") (Lanzino, Rabinstein, & Brown, 2009).

Diagnosis

Auscultation should be part of the routine physical examination of patients with risk factors for vascular disease. Although carotid bruits have limited value for the diagnosis of carotid artery stenosis, they are good markers of generalized atherosclerosis. The presence of a carotid bruit is associated with increased risk of vascular disease including stroke, myocardial infarction, and cardiovascular death (Lanzino, Rabinstein, & Brown, 2009).

For asymptomatic patients with vascular risk factors, carotid auscultation is a sufficient screening test. However, for patients with symptoms of transient ischemic attack (TIA) or stroke, the evaluation for carotid artery disease cannot be limited to auscultation of the neck because carotid bruits have relatively low sensitivity for the detection of moderate or severe carotid artery stenosis. Specificity is good for carotid artery disease in general, but it is actually lower for greater degrees of stenosis. Because bruits are generated by turbulent flow, they may be strong with mild stenosis and may even disappear when the stenosis becomes critical and causes marked restriction of flow. Therefore, symptomatic patients must be evaluated with imaging studies (Lanzino, Rabinstein, & Brown, 2009).

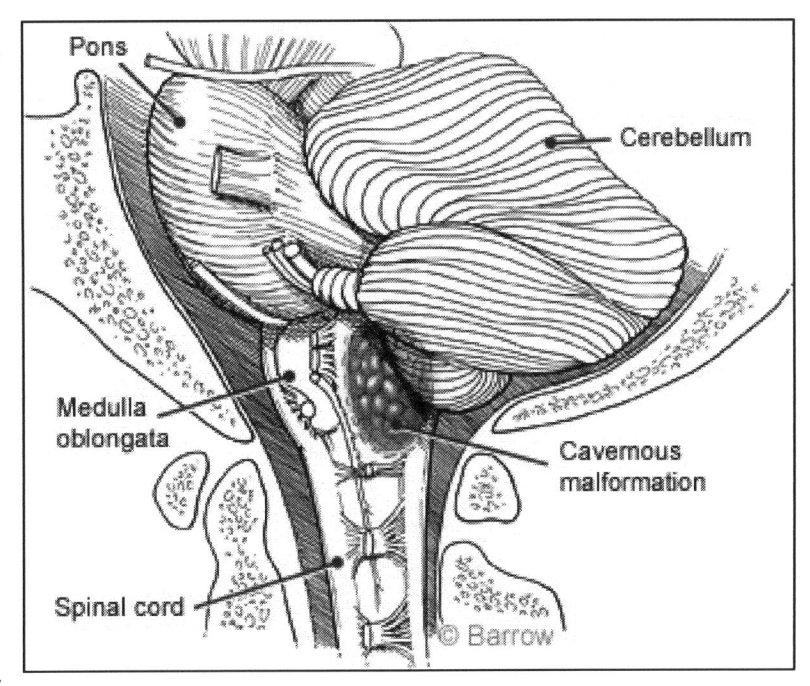

The definition of hemodynamically significant carotid artery stenosis is based on data from the RCTs on CEA. Exact quantification of the degree of stenosis is crucial in selecting proper treatment. This quantification is particularly important for patients with asymptomatic carotid artery stenosis because of the marginal benefit they receive from surgery. Doppler ultrasonography, which is readily available and noninvasive, is usually the first diagnostic imaging tool used to screen for carotid artery stenosis. However, it is highly dependent on operator experience and skill. When compared with catheter angiography, Doppler ultrasonography has a sensitivity of 86% and a specificity of 87% for the detection of hemodynamically significant carotid artery stenosis (Lanzino, Rabinstein, & Brown, 2009).

Catheter angiography is the criterion standard for defining the degree of stenosis and the morphologic features of the offending plaque. However, catheter angiography is neither feasible nor recommended in every patient because of its risks and costs. Computed tomographic angiography and magnetic resonance angiography have gained popularity for use in the diagnosis of carotid artery stenosis, often replacing conventional catheter angiography. In our practice, magnetic resonance angiography or computed tomographic angiography is used as a confirmatory test after results of a Doppler study suggest hemodynamically significant stenosis in an asymptomatic patient. Among symptomatic patients, a Doppler study is completed as part of the emergency evaluation of every patient with TIA or stroke. If a patient is considered for invasive treatment, these angiographic techniques are subsequently performed for improved definition of the stenosis. Invasive treatment is considered for symptomatic patients with stenosis greater than 50% and for asymptomatic patients with stenosis greater than 60% (Lanzino, Rabinstein, & Brown, 2009).

Cavernous Angiomas

A cerebral cavernous malformation (also known as cavernous angioma or cavernous hemangioma) is an abnormal group of small blood vessels that may be found in the brain and spinal cord. These lesions can be quiet for many years; however, they can manifest themselves by bleeding. Cerebral cavernous malformations may cause serious neurological symptoms, and even death can occur as a result of severe bleeding or pressure on the brain or nerves.

Symptoms

- Seizures
- Headaches
- Paralysis
- Cerebral hemorrhage
- Seizures may be controlled with anti-epileptic drugs.
- Surgery may be necessary to remove a cerebral cavernous malformation that is causing symptoms or that suffered multiple bleedings (University of Pittsburg Medical Center, 2013).

Diagnosis

- Tests for diagnosing a cerebral cavernous malformation
- Cerebral cavernous malformations can be diagnosed by imaging studies such as CT and MRI scans.

Treatments

- Anti-epileptic drugs are typically given to control seizures. However, surgery may be required to remove the malformation if it is causing recurrent bleeding or other dangerous symptoms.
- Surgery
- MRI
- High Definition Fiber Tracking (HDFT)
- MEG
- Gamma Knife® radiosurgery
  - Gamma Knife radiosurgery is a painless procedure that uses hundreds of highly focused radiation beams to target tumors and lesions within the brain with no surgical incision ("Cerebral cavernous malformation," 2013).

Carotid Dissection

Hemorrhage within the carotid artery; intimal tear results in communication of intravascular blood and direct connection with the vessel wall cavity; development of intramural hematoma without direct connection with the vessel lumen (Bader & Littlejohns, 2004).

Epidemiology

- Dissections responsible for 1-2.5% of ischemic strokes in general population; responsible for 5-20% of strokes in individuals younger than 45 years of age
- Average annual incidence of spontaneous cervical dissection was 2.6 per 100,000
- Age, sex, race
    - All ages affected; occurs more frequently between the ages of 35 and 50 years
    - Males and females affected equally
    - Intracranial dissection occurs more often in males
    - No racial preponderance
- Types of dissections
    - Traumatic-non-penetrating injury
    - Spontaneous (Bader & Littlejohns, 2004)

Etiology

- Sudden severe stretch of ICA over upper cervical spine; hyperextended, lateral flexion to opposite side due to chiropractic neck manipulations, sports, coughing or sneezing, motor vehicle accidents, falls, sexual activity, strangulation/hanging, or direct blow to artery
- Direct compression between angle of mandible and upper cervical spine
- Blunt trauma
- Endarterectomy
- Arteriopathies: fibromuscular dysplasia occurs in up to 15% of cases; extreme vessel tortuosity; Ehlers-Danlos syndrome; Marfan's syndrome (Bader & Littlejohns, 2004)

Mechanism of Symptom Development

- Subintimal hematoma
    - Luminal stenosis causing distal ischemia from low flow
    - May lead to stroke, TIA, or no symptoms
    - Symptoms dependent on adequacy of collateral supply
    - Symptoms may wax/wane with BP changes
- Subintimal/subadventitial
    - Exposure of basement membrane
    - Leads to platelet aggregation
    - Possible recurrent embolization (Bader & Littlejohns, 2004)

Assessment

- Subjective
    - Pain: hallmark feature of presentation
        - Ipsilateral head, neck, or scalp areas

- - - Sharp, throbbing
  - Ischemic symptoms
    - Amarousis fugax; transient monocular blindness; TIA or stroke
- Objective
  - Ipsilateral partial Horner's syndrome
    - Due to disruption of sympathetic fibers located along wall of ICA
    - Presents with ptosis and miosis; facial sweat preserved as innervation of sweat gland is along ECA
    - Ipsilateral CN phases IX, X, XI, XII
    - Audible bruit
- Diagnosis
  - Conventional angiography
  - MRI
  - MRA
  - CT
  - CTA
  - Carotid ultrasound
  - TCD (Bader & Littlejohns, 2004)

DISSECTED INTERNAL CAROTID ARTERY

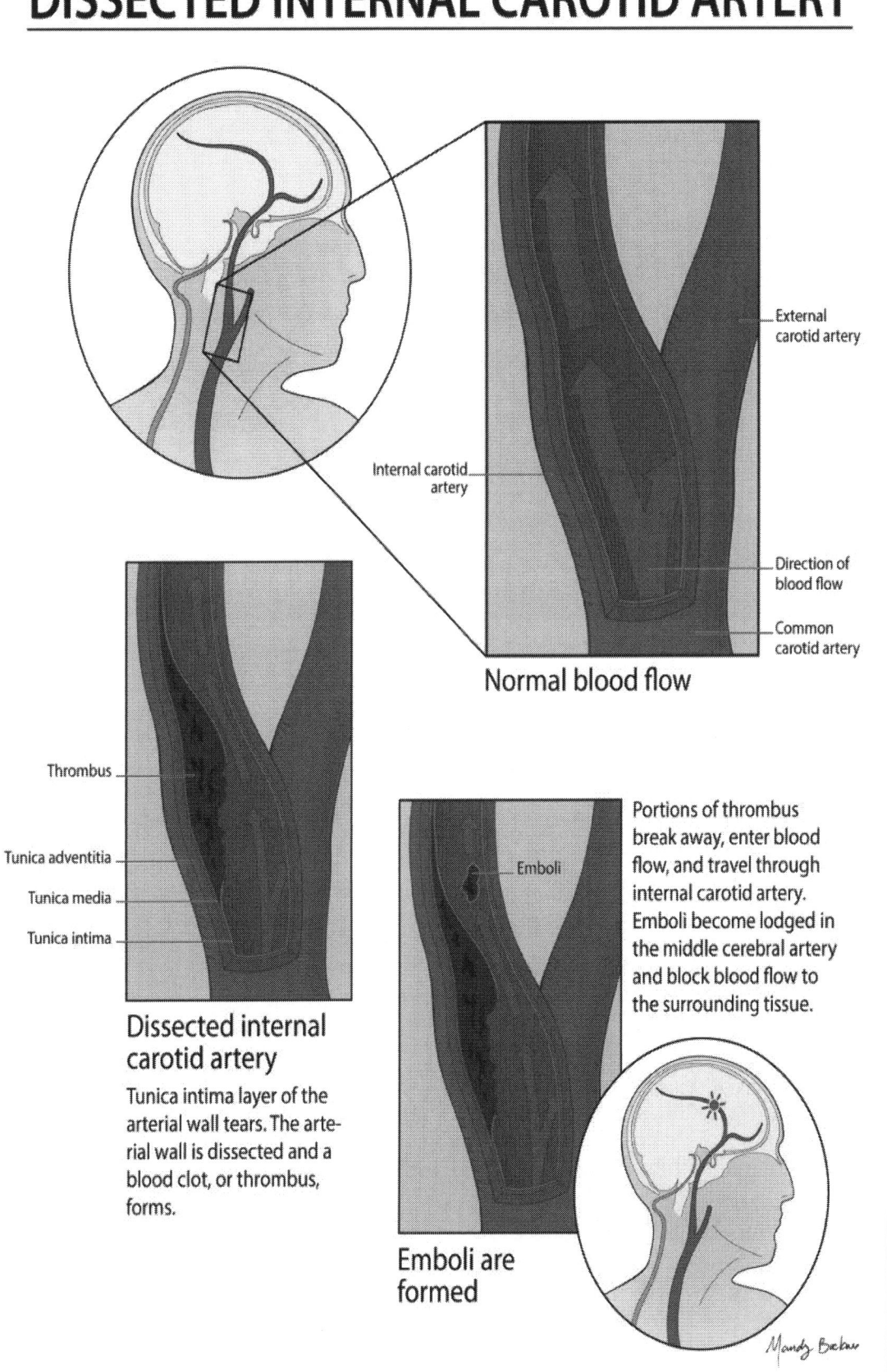

Normal blood flow

- External carotid artery
- Internal carotid artery
- Direction of blood flow
- Common carotid artery

Dissected internal carotid artery

- Thrombus
- Tunica adventitia
- Tunica media
- Tunica intima

Tunica intima layer of the arterial wall tears. The arterial wall is dissected and a blood clot, or thrombus, forms.

Emboli are formed

Emboli

Portions of thrombus break away, enter blood flow, and travel through internal carotid artery. Emboli become lodged in the middle cerebral artery and block blood flow to the surrounding tissue.

Treatment

- Medical
    - Anticoagulation for prevention of embolization for three to six months
        - Contraindicated in dissections complicated by SAH
        - Heparin: IV infusion; therapeutic target PTT 1.5 to 2.0 times control
        - Antiplatelet agents: Aspirin, dosage range 81 to 1300 mg orally per day; limited use; primarily when anticoagulation is limited
    - Surgery (for patients refractory to medical management)
        - Bypass procedures
    - Endovascular procedures
        - Angioplasty and stenting
        - Vessel occlusion with embolization, coiling, or litigations
    - Nursing care is same as with ischemic stroke (Bader & Littlejohns, 2004)

Ischemic Stroke

An ischemic stroke is defined as a *dramatic* development of a focal neurological deficit caused by an interruption of blood flow to the brain. Blood flow is impaired because of a blockage to one or more of the arteries supplying blood to the brain. The process leading to this blockage is known as thrombosis. Strokes caused in this way are called thrombotic strokes. Thrombosis generally occurs in deep vessels. Much large vessel thrombosis is caused by a combination of pre-existing atherosclerosis followed by rapid blood clot formation. Thrombotic stroke patients often have underlying coronary artery disease, and myocardial infarction is a frequent cause of death in thrombotic stroke patients (Bader & Littlejohns, 2004).

Epidemiology

- 750,000 new strokes annually
- 3rd leading cause of death in the U.S.
- Leading cause of adult disability
- 90% of survivors will have some type of deficit

Etiology

Ischemic strokes are associated with modifiable and non-modifiable risk factors
- Non-modifiable
    - Age: there is an increased risk in adults >55 years old; risk doubles each decade after 55 years; one quarter of stroke victims are younger than 65 years of age
    - Sex: 9% greater incidence in men; 61% of stroke deaths occur in women
    - Race: African-Americans have twice the risk of death and disability
    - Prior stroke: 3-10% recurrence within first 30 days; 4-14% recurrence within the first year
    - Family history (Bader & Littlejohns, 2004)

- o Modifiable risk factors
  - o HTN: BP >140/60 mm Hg
  - o Hypercholesterolemia: LDL target goal is <100 mg/dl
  - o Diabetes Mellitus: hyperglycemia accelerates atherosclerosis; hyperinsulinemia increases risk
  - o Hypercoagulopathy: related to cancer, pregnancy, high RBCs, sickle cell anemia
  - o Cardiac disease: CAD and CHF double risk; MI increases risk, Atrial fibrillation; patent foramen ovale; carotid artery disease
- o Modifiable Behavioral
  - o Smoking
  - o ETOH
  - o Smoking while taking oral contraceptives
  - o Sedentary lifestyle
  - o Obesity
  - o Drug use
  - o Stress (Bader & Littlejohns, 2004)

Prevention

A majority of strokes can be prevented by the control of primary, secondary, and lifestyle risk factors:
- o HTN - Maintain SBP < 140 mm Hg and DBP < 90 mm Hg; monitor in prehypertension (130-139 mm Hg/80-89 mm Hg)
- o Control cholesterol levels through diet, exercise, and statin agents
- o A. fib - Daily Aspirin or Coumadin
- o Hyperglycemia - Target blood glucose <140 mg/dl (BP goal in DM <130 mm Hg)

Pathophysiology

An ischemic stroke can occur in two ways: embolic or thrombotic. These lesions form during periods of inactivity. Atherosclerotic plaques in the carotid occur inside the injured vessel. Inflammation within the vessel causes platelet aggregation. Coagulation occurs at the site of injury, and a thrombus/small emboli forms. This leads to decreased blood flow through the carotids, leaving collateral circulation.

Criteria for Stroke Treatment with tPA

- Inclusion:
  - o Clinical diagnosis of stroke with significant, non-resolving deficit
  - o Age > 18 years
  - o < 3-hour window from last known to be neurologically intact
  - o ICU level of care must be available
  - o Non-contrast CT scan without evidence of hemorrhage

- Contraindications
  - History:
    - History of CNS hemorrhage, aneurysm, or AV Malformation
    - Seizure at stroke onset
    - Ongoing acute MI
    - Recent arterial puncture at non-compressible site
    - No lumbar puncture within last seven days
    - Major surgery or trauma within 14 days
    - GI/GU bleed within 21 days
    - Lactation or pregnancy within last 30 days
    - Head trauma, bleed, surgery, or stroke within last three months
  - Vital signs:
    - SBP >185, DBP >110
  - Lab Analysis:
    - Platelets < 100,000
    - Treated with heparin within 48 hours
    - INR >7.1
    - Blood glucose <50 or >400

Embolic Stroke - Small emboli form and travel from other areas of the body and lodge in the cerebral vessels (Hayden Gephart, 2013).

Lacunar Stroke - Thrombosis of small penetrating arteries.

- Often related to HTN and lipohyalinosis
- Affects arms, legs, and face; however, deficits are equal
- Motor - pure hemiparesis if perforators to pons or internal capsule are affected (Hayden Gephart, 2013)
- Sensory - if perforators to thalamus or posterior limb of internal capsule, then patient will present with pure hemisensory deficits (Hayden Gephart, 2013)

Hemorrhagic Stroke - Cerebral arteries prone to hemorrhage because they lack elastic laminae (from HTN).

- Mostly affects basal ganglia, pons, and thalamus because perforators branch directly from high-pressure arteries.
- Related to CV malformation, vasculitis, amyloidosis, drug use (cocaine, methamphetamines), collagen/vascular disorders, prior stroke, neoplasm, and anticoagulation.

Intracerebral Hemorrhage (ICH)

ICH is bleeding within the brain parenchyma that can result from trauma or occur spontaneously (non-traumatic). Hemorrhage is different than *a hematoma*. A hematoma is defined as the localized extravasation of blood within the tissues; a hemorrhage refers to the actual event in which the blood escapes from its normal confines within the vessels (Bader & Littlejohns, 2004).

Epidemiology

- 10-20% of all strokes are a result of an ICH
- High incidence of mortality in these patients (30 days after an ICH, mortality was 43%)
- 12% of survivors will have a mild disability
- Incidence is related to age and race
    o Occurs in 2 per 100,000 people younger than 35 years of age
    o Occurs in 350 per 100,000 people older than 80 years of age
    o More common in young and middle-aged African-Americans than in Caucasians (Bader & Littlejohns, 2004)

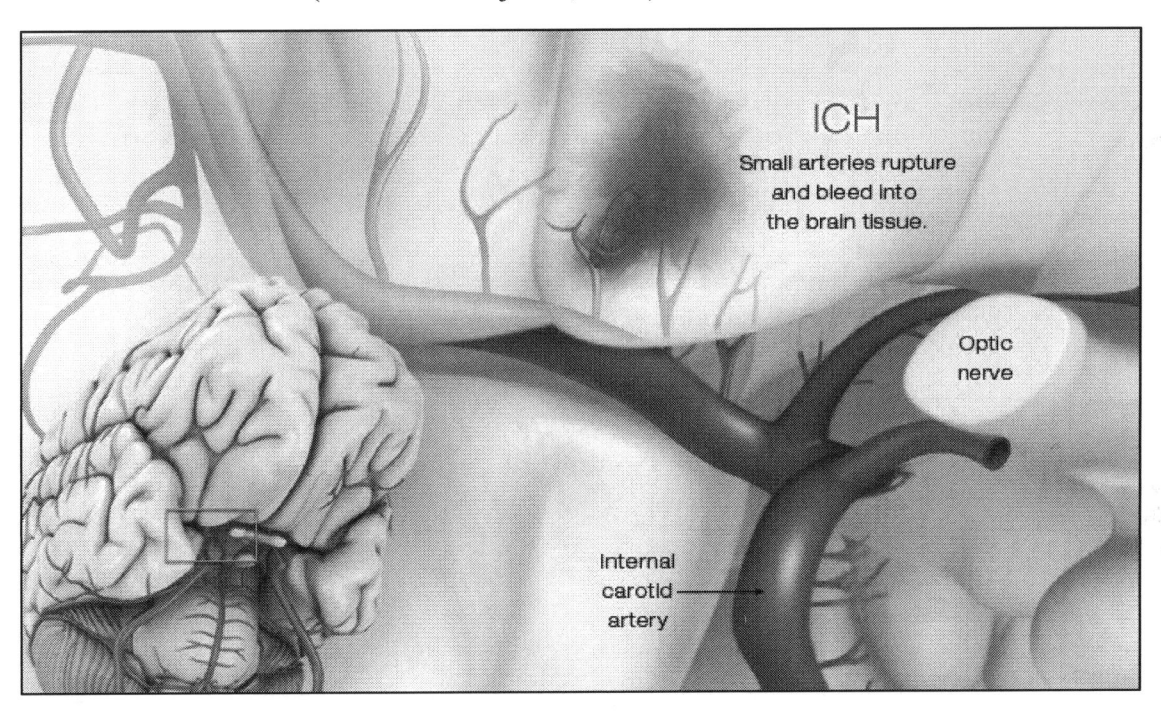

Etiology

- Hypertension – 56-81% of cases; chronic HTN leads to deterioration of blood vessels
- Vascular malformations - AV malformations; post-operative resections
- Cavernous malformations - Low flow, low pressure vascular lesions made up of a group of dilated capillaries
- Charcot-Bouchard microaneurysms - Bifurcation of small, perforating branches of lateral lenticulostriate arteries in the basal ganglia
- Brain tumor - Usually malignant Glioblastoma, lymphoma, metastatic tumors
- Venous infarction (sagittal sinus syndrome)
- Vasculitis

- Drug abuse - Cocaine, amphetamines, and opioids (Bader & Littlejohns, 2004)

Presentation

- Seizures most common in supratentorial lesions
- Focal deficits seen in patients with brainstem and spinal cord abnormalities
- Often discovered during evaluation of non-specific symptoms such as headache (Bader & Littlejohns, 2004)

Assessment

- Subjective data - sudden onset of focal neurological deficits that progress over minutes to hours; headache, nausea, vomiting, and decreased LOC
- Objective data
    - History - HTN, prior ICH, known cerebral vascular malformations, anticoagulant therapy
    - Physical exam - severe HA, decreased LOC, hemiplegia, paresis on arm and/or leg; numbness/tingling in arm and/or leg; CN abnormalities-unequal pupils with loss of pupillary reaction; disconjugate gaze, facial weakness, swallowing problems; aphasia, extinction, gaze preference
- Diagnostic data
    - CT is most important part of the initial evaluation
        - Identifies acute hemorrhage size and location
        - Reveals potential emergent clinical situation
    - MRI can detect structural abnormalities like AVMs and specific tumor sites and can give more details about course of problem
        - Contraindicated in those who are morbidly obese, have implantable medical devices, or have orbital injuries
    - CTA
        - Noninvasive; can detect arterial structural abnormalities of the head and neck
        - Requires peripheral, large-bore access
        - Shorter test (20 minutes) compared to MRI (40 minutes)
    - Cerebral angiogram
        - Invasive, but "gold standard;" high-resolution method to visualize cerebral vasculature
        - Ideal for diagnosing aneurysms or AVMs
        - Patients with iodine sensitivity require steroid premedication
    - Laboratory Test
        - CBC, Sedimentation rate
            - Elevated WBCs may be indicative of infection
            - Evaluates inflammatory processes as cause
        - PT, activated PTT, and INR
            - Evaluates for coagulopathy
            - Evaluates whether INR is supratherapeutic

- Electrolytes
- Electrocardiogram
  - Evaluates for vegetations on heart valves
  - Assesses for endocarditis as source of hemorrhage (mycotic aneurysm)
- Chest X-ray (Bader & Littlejohns, 2004)

Patient Problems/Interventions

- Increased ICP – focal motor/sensory deficits and/or decline in LOC and diagnostic imaging demonstrates acute ICH
  o Emergent workup
    - initial airway stabilization; intubation/mechanical ventilation for GCS score 3 to 8
    - establish IV access (2 sites, large bore); Normal saline; labs
    - Foley catheter
    - emergent CT scan of brain without contrast
    - orders to keep SBP <170 mm Hg with IV Labetalol or sodium nitroprusside (Nipride)
  o Non-operative management - appropriate if hematoma <20 ml or for patients who are minimally symptomatic (GCS score >12)
  o Assess airway and maintain oxygenation/ventilation with supplemental oxygen
  o Manage BP - parameters depend on patient's history of HTN, ICP issues, and presumed cause of hemorrhage
    - Treat more aggressively in patients with ischemic stroke
    - Goals are SBP 150 to 170 mm Hg and mean arterial pressure ≤130 mm Hg
    - Labetalol 5 to 10 mg intermittent bolus to a total of 300 mg
    - Esmolol 500 micrograms/kg loading does the 50 to 200 micrograms/kg/minute
    - Nitroprusside 0.5 to 10 micrograms/kg/min
    - Hydralazine every four to six hours
    - Enalapril 0.625 to 1.2 mg every six hours or as determined otherwise
    - Avoid hypotension - administer NeoSynephrine or Dopamine if required
    - IVFs with NS; avoid glucose solutions
    - Monitor labs as per order
    - Correct bleeding/coagulopathy
      - Fresh frozen plasma
      - Vitamin K for endogenous clotting factor
    - Phenytoin is preferred prophylaxis against seizures (1 g loading dose, then 100 mg TID to maintain therapeutic level of 10 to 20)
    - Swallow evaluation when appropriate
    - DVT prophylaxis (SCDs, compression hose) (Bader & Littlejohns, 2004)

- Patients with symptomatic hemorrhage (GCS score 3 to 11) and decision for aggressive management
    - ABCs, support with mechanical ventilation/intubation (avoid hyperventilation)
    - ICP management - place ventriculostomy/brain oxygen monitors
        - Maintain CPP (MAP-ICP) >60 mm Hg
        - Insert small-bore feeding tube or NG tube and start early enteral nutrition
- Conservative management - large hemorrhages in dominant hemisphere means remote chance of good outcome or poor neurological examination
    - Determine if patient has executed advanced directives
    - Provide comfort care as indicated
- Surgical (indications are poorly defined)
    - Associated mass effect, shift of midline structures
    - Evacuation of hematoma can reduce ICP
    - Unclear data on patient outcome (Bader & Littlejohns, 2004)

Nursing Interventions

- Critical care - all of these patients will be admitted to the intensive care unit (ICU) for hourly monitoring of neurological status and vital signs
- Acute care - continued observation of neurological examination; BP management; continue PT, OT, ST; begin discharge planning; consider rehabilitation services
- Rehabilitation - primary focus is restorative to improve mobility, ADLs, and bowel/bladder management; teach family about assistive devices, swallowing precautions, and toileting
- Post-hospitalization - the PCP should provide ongoing monitoring and management of HTN; counsel patient and family on importance of follow up and compliance (Bader & Littlejohns, 2004)

Prevention

- Control hypertension in order to reduce the incidence of recurrent hemorrhage
- Reduction or cessation of cocaine and alcohol abuse
- Monitor INR frequently in patients on anticoagulants (higher risk if INR > 3) (Bader & Littlejohns, 2004)

Subarachnoid Hemorrhage

Subarachnoid hemorrhage is bleeding in the area between the brain and the thin tissues that cover the brain. This area is called the subarachnoid space (Bader & Littlejohns, 2004).

Causes

Subarachnoid hemorrhage can be caused by:

- Bleeding from an arteriovenous malformation (AVM)
- Bleeding disorder
- Bleeding from a cerebral aneurysm
- Head injury
- Unknown cause (idiopathic)
- Anticoagulant therapy
- Subarachnoid hemorrhage caused by injury is often seen in the elderly who have fallen and suffered head trauma. Among the young, the most common injury leading to subarachnoid hemorrhage is motor vehicle crashes.

Risks

- Aneurysm in other blood vessels
- Fibromuscular dysplasia (FMD) and other connective tissue disorders
- High blood pressure
- History of polycystic kidney disease
- Smoking
- Strong family history of aneurysms may increase risk (Bader & Littlejohns, 2004)

Symptoms

The main symptom is a *severe headache* that starts suddenly (often called a thunderclap headache). It is often worse near the back of the head. Many people often describe it as the "worst headache ever" and unlike any other type of headache pain. The headache may start after a popping or snapping feeling in the head.

- Decreased consciousness and alertness
- Eye discomfort in bright light (photophobia)
- Mood and personality changes including confusion and irritability
- Muscle aches (especially neck and shoulder pain)
- Nausea and vomiting
- Numbness in part of the body
- Seizure
- Stiff neck
- Vision problems including double vision, blind spots, and temporary vision loss in one eye

Assessment

- A physical exam may show a stiff neck
- A brain and nervous system exam may show signs of decreased nerve and brain function (focal neurologic deficit)
- An eye exam may show decreased eye movements - a sign of damage to the cranial nerves (in milder cases, no problems may be seen on an eye exam) (Hayden Gephart, 2013)

Diagnostic Procedures

- Cerebral angiography of blood vessels of the brain
- CT scan angiography (using contrast dye)
- Transcranial Doppler ultrasound - assess blood flow in the arteries of the brain
- MRI and MRA

Treatment

- Medication to control blood pressure
- Nimodipine to prevent artery spams
- Analgesics and anti-anxiety medications to relieve headache and reduce pressure in the skull
- Phenytoin or other medications to prevent or treat seizures
- Stool softeners or laxatives to prevent straining during bowel movements
- Avoid suddenly changing position (Bader & Littlejohns, 2004)

Goals of Treatment

- Preserve life and fullest functional potential
- Treat the cause of bleeding
- Relieve symptoms
- Prevent complications such as permanent brain damage (stroke)

Surgical Treatment

- Remove large collections of blood or relieve pressure on the brain if the hemorrhage is due to an injury
- Repair the aneurysm if the hemorrhage is due to an aneurysm rupture
- If the patient is critically ill, surgery may have to wait until the person is more stable.
- Craniotomy (burr hole) and aneurysm-clipping to close the aneurysm
- Endovascular coiling - placing coils in the aneurysm and stents in the blood vessel to cage the coils reduces the risk of further bleeding
- If no aneurysm is found, the patient should be closely watched by a healthcare team and may need more imaging tests.

Treatment for Coma

- Draining tube placed in the brain to relieve pressure
- Life support
- Methods to protect the airway
- Special positioning

Nursing Interventions

- Promote environment that is non-stimulating, quiet, and comfortable
- Maintain patient on bed - rest with toilet privileges or as required
- Visitors should be limited
- Assist with activities of daily living
- Ensure anti-embolic stockings are worn or a calf-compression device is used to reduce the incidence of deep-venous thrombosis

Intraventricular Hemorrhage

Intraventricular hemorrhage (IVH) is known as bleeding into the fluid-filled areas (ventricles) inside the brain. The condition occurs most often in premature babies (Lee, 2013).

Epidemiology

Brain hemorrhage has the highest morbidity and mortality rate of any stroke subtype. Intracerebral hemorrhage (ICH) and subarachnoid hemorrhage (SAH) account for about 15% and 5% of the 750,000 strokes that occur every year in the U.S., totaling more than 45,000 patients per year (Holly, Hanley, & Ziai, 2011).

Pathophysiology

- Primary IVH is confined to the ventricular system, arising from an intraventricular source or a lesion contiguous to the ventricles.
- Examples include intraventricular trauma, aneurysm, vascular malformation, and tumor usually involving the choroid plexus.
- Approximately 70% of IVHs are secondary; secondary IVHs may occur as an extension of an intraparenchymal hemorrhage or SAH into the ventricular system.
- Risk factors for IVH include old age, higher baseline ICH volume, mean arterial pressure values greater than 120 mm Hg, and location of the primary lesion (Holly, Hanley, & Ziai, 2011).

Prognosis

- Blood in the ventricular system contributes to morbidity in a variety of ways.
- Damage to the reticular activating system and thalamus during the acute phase of hemorrhage expansion causes a decreased level of consciousness.
- Coma appears to be prolonged with both a larger volume of blood in the ventricles and a longer exposure.
- Ventricular blood clots blocking cerebrospinal fluid (CSF) conduits cause acute obstructive hydrocephalus, an immediate life-threatening condition limiting cerebral perfusion and potentially contributing to mass effect and resultant cerebral edema.

- The inflammatory reaction caused by blood breakdown products in the ventricles also may affect long-term cognitive function independent of clot volume or mass effect, as demonstrated in experimental IVH (Holly, Hanley, & Ziai, 2011).

Emergency Care

- A depressed level of consciousness may lead to loss of neurologic reflexes protecting a patent airway, placing the patient at risk for hypoxia, hypercapnia, and aspiration.
- If endotracheal intubation and mechanical ventilation are required, sedatives and neuromuscular blocking agents that do not elevate intracranial pressure (ICP) should be selected.
- Overaggressive treatment of blood pressure may decrease cerebral perfusion pressure and promote focal ischemia adjacent to hematoma.
    - Treat systolic blood pressure (SBP) greater than 180 mm Hg or diastolic blood pressure greater than 105 mm Hg
    - Target SBP goals ≥ 160 mm Hg are associated with hematoma enlargement compared with SBP goals ≤ 150 mm Hg
- Coagulopathy is associated with ICH and should be corrected as quickly as possible.
    - Fresh frozen plasma infusion followed by oral vitamin K should be given without delay in the emergency department to manage warfarin-related ICH (Holly, Hanley, & Ziai, 2011).

Intensive Care Unit Care

- Patients with IVH will require care in the intensive care unit (ICU) setting.
- Patients should have the benefit of conventional neurologic ICU care including resuscitation with intravenous fluids.
- Placement of the head of bed at 30°
- Correction of fever with antipyretics
- Deep-venous thrombosis prophylaxis with sequential compression devices and/or compression stockings
- Low-dose prophylactic anticoagulation should be initiated 48 hours after injury (Holly, Hanley, & Ziai, 2011).

Nursing Interventions

- Seizure prevention
    - Clinical and electrographic seizures should be aggressively treated, but anti-epileptic drug (AED) prophylaxis is more controversial.
    - Frequently, AEDs are used prophylactically in ICH to avoid seizure-associated neurologic deterioration and re-bleeding.
    - Phenytoin is the AED gold standard (Holly, Hanley, & Ziai, 2011).

- Prevent hematoma expansion
  o Hematoma growth is an independent determinant of both mortality and functional outcome after ICH (Holly, Hanley, & Ziai, 2011).
- Management of intracranial pressure
  o Intraventricular catheter (IVC)
  o External ventricular drain (EVD)
- Manage intraventricular thrombolysis
  o Ventriculostomy appears to be effective in controlling ICP, but this technique does little to reduce morbidity and does not address the *inflammatory* process
  o Intraventricular rt-PA
- Prepare patient for surgical evacuation
  o Although the conventional treatment is ventricular drainage, open craniotomy, and/or surgical evacuation of IVH, stereotactic drainage of IVH and minimally invasive treatments have limited exposure in the literature (Holly, Hanley, & Ziai, 2011).

Headaches

Perhaps one of the most debilitating disorders, headaches are experienced by healthy patients and the chronically ill. Although pain is subjective, most can relate to the nuisance that such a disorder can be. Headaches can be a symptom of a minor problem or indicative of a life-threatening medical emergency. Headache encompasses a range of symptoms with a broad etiology. The two classifications of headaches are:
- *Primary headache* - characterized by pain *without* abnormal pathophysiology
  o Migraine
  o Tension-type headache
  o Cluster headache and paroxysmal headache
  o Miscellaneous headaches not associated with structural lesion
- *Secondary headache* - pain due to underlying abnormality including, but not limited to, intracranial lesion, abscess, or tumor; intracranial bleed from trauma, arteriovenous malformation, or aneurysm; infection; increased intracranial pressure; craniofacial neuralgias; and disorder of the eyes, ears, sinus, and teeth
  o May also be associated with substances or their withdrawal (rebound headache) (Bader & Littlejohns, 2004)

Epidemiology

Incidence: (data may not reflect a large amount of the population that does not report headaches, but do suffer)
- Annually, 90% of men and 95% of women will have some type of headache
- Annually, 23 million Americans have episodes of migraines
- 42% of women and 36% of men suffer tension-type headaches

Age/gender relativity
- Before puberty, a higher incidence in males than in females
- By adolescence, incidence increase in females and decrease in males

- Incidence in females increases from teens to 40s, then tapers off (Bader & Littlejohns, 2004)

Etiology/Contributing Factors

- *Migraine threshold*: if high, a person rarely or never suffers a migraine. If low, even the mildest triggers can bring on an attack.
- *Threshold*, or level of susceptibility to migraine, is genetically determined; heterogeneous and linked to more than one gene or gene location.
- Genetic link for familial hemiplegic migraine on chromosome 19
- There is a strong familial risk for migraine; close to 70% of patients have a family history of migraines.
- *Comorbidity*: people with migraines seem to have a higher incidence of other conditions
    - Epilepsy
    - Anxiety and/or depression
    - Stroke (migraine with aura)
    - Comorbidities may influence treatment (Bader & Littlejohns, 2004)

Pathophysiology

- Migraine is believed to be a genetically influenced neurobiological disorder
- Threshold is exceeded through a combination of stress, environmental, and hormonal factors
- Persistent headaches lower the threshold further, leading to recurrent or persistent (status migraine) episodes of pain with minimal provocation.
- Interaction of neurotransmitter and receptor function activates pain pathways and decreases pain modulation
    - Migraine "generator" is thought to be housed in the brainstem in region that connects to the spinal tract of the trigeminal nerve
    - Activation of the trigeminal system results in a release of neuropeptides: Substance P, Calcitonin gene-related peptide, and Neurokinin A
    - These neuropeptides cause neurogenic sterile inflammation and increase vascular permeability and local dilation of blood vessel, causing pain syndrome via the trigeminal pathway.
    - Pain is felt anywhere throughout the head that is innervated by the trigeminal system
        - Pain may be unilateral, temporal, throbbing, or may start at the base of the skull or above and below the eyes
    - Serotonin levels in the brain are thought to be related to migraine (Bader & Littlejohns, 2004)

Assessment

- *Subjective* - diagnosis is made in large by patient history; use of intake questionnaire is a helpful and efficient way to obtain

- Onset of headaches (years, months, new onset)
- Location (unilateral, bilateral, migratory, global)
- Quality of pain (sharp, throbbing, dull, achy, etc.)
- Severity of pain - pain scale, duration
- Frequency of headache
- Description of each type of headache suffered
- Associated symptoms
- Presence of an aura (transitory neurological symptom preceding a headache; <60 minutes)
    - Visual scatoma, flashing lights, visual distortions
    - Paresthesias of the extremities or around the mouth
- Identify factors that trigger
    - Dietary: MSG, dairy, yeast, tyramine, caffeine, chocolate
    - Alcohol, especially red wine
    - Emotional factors: anxiety, stress, emotional letdown
    - Sleep: too little, too much
    - Hormonal fluctuations
    - Medication: estrogen, nitroglycerine, ranitidine, others
    - Environmental: weather, barometric change, odors, fluorescent lights, sound
- Patient's lifestyle regarding exercise, rest, meal patterns, anxiety, stress, tobacco and alcohol use, and caffeine intake
- History of head injury including MVCs
- Medication history including OTCs, herbs, birth control, all medications
- General medical history
- Family history

- *Objective*
    - Physical exam: generally normal (unless patient is having an *acute*, complicated migraine)
    - Abnormal findings may include:
        - Temporal artery tenderness (temporal arteritis)
        - Occipital nerve tenderness (occipital neuralgia)
        - Temporal mandibular joint tenderness
        - Neck and back muscle tenderness, myofascial tenderness (muscle contraction headache, cervical strain) (Bader & Littlejohns, 2004)

Diagnostics

- Laboratory evaluation
    - Sedimentation rate (temporal arteritis)
    - C-reactive protein
    - Thyroid profile (looking for hypothyroidism)
- Imaging considered for:
    - *Thunderclap headache*: very acute onset; severe pain (r/o aneurysm)
    - *Worst headache of my life*: rule out aneurysm
    - Headache associated with fever, stiff neck (rule out meningitis)

- Headache associated with severe vomiting or projectile vomiting (rule out aneurysm)
- New onset of headache after age 50 (less common for headaches to start in that age group; rule out tumor)
- A patient experiencing cognitive, abnormal neurological exam or papilledema
- A patient with cancer or HIV (rule out metastatic lesion, abscess, and infection)
- CT scan: best for acute injury to rule out bleed
- MRI: use to rule out space-occupying lesion, demyelinating lesions, ischemia, abscess; more sensitive than CT
- MRA: use to rule out vascular abnormality, aneurysm
- Lumbar puncture: use to rule out meningitis
- EEG: use if intermittent neurological symptoms suggest possible seizure activity (may be difficult to differentiate aura from seizures) (Bader & Littlejohns, 2004)

Patient Problems

- Pain with mild to moderate headache
    - Tension-type headaches described as "pressing," "squeezing," "band around head," or "hat too tight;" pain is most often bilateral or global, not throbbing, pulsing, or disabling; is not exacerbated by physical activity
    - *Treatment*
        - NSAIDs
        - Butabital, caffeine, and aspirin or acetaminophen combination such as Esgic, Fiorinal, or Fioricet
        - Isometheptene (Midrin)
        - Muscle relaxants such as carisoprodol (Soma), cyclobenzaprine (Flexiril), or tizanidine (Zanaflex)
        - Nursing: typically in outpatient setting, acute, and chronic care
            - OTC analgesics
            - Local measures including heat, cold, or massage, particularly if there is neck and upper back pain and stiffness
            - Relaxation exercises
            - Referral for chiropractic treatment or physical therapy
- Headache associated with moderate to severe pain (migraine) or acute or abortive treatment
    - Migraine headaches are described as episodic, disabling headaches, or with or without auras; pain is pulsing or throbbing and moderate to severe; pain is unilateral, bilateral, and is worsened by physical activity
        - Headache associated with nasal symptoms or "sinus" may in fact be migraines.
        - Most effective treatment for disabling migraine is using the *triptan* class of drugs:
            - They work in the CNS to constrict vessels, decrease substance P, and decrease trigeminal nerve inflammation (Axert, Relepax, Frova, Amerge, Maxalt, Imitrex, Zomig)

- Side effects of triptans are somnolence; asthenia; parasthesias; tingling; sensation of tightness in throat; flushing of upper chest, neck, and face; and dizziness
- Contraindicated in patients with CAD, HTN, or multiple cardiac risk factors
- Ergot alkaloids, which are *nonselective agonists*, are ergotamine oral and suppository (Cafergot) and dihydroergotamine (DHE) parenteral and nasal spray (Migranal)
    - Side effects: nausea, dizziness, paresthesias, abdominal cramps, chest tightness, and significant arterial constrictions
    - Should NOT be given within 24 hours of triptan administration
- Adjunctive medications: Chlorpromazine and prochlorperazine (IV, PO, PR) relieve associated nausea and vomiting and relieve pain centrally. Metoclopramide can be used for n/v and slowed peristalsis. Parenteral diphenhydramine may improve pain control. Adding NSAIDs to triptan may improve pain relief.
- Narcotics are not routinely used in the treatment of headache, but may be prescribed if other medications are not effective. Codeine or meperidine may be used with caution during pregnancy.
- To break a prolonged attack and intractable pain, give DHE IV or SC with an antiemetic, valproate sodium IV (Depacon), or methylprednisolone (Solu-medrol) IV
- Pain associated with very rapid onset and excruciating headache
    o Cluster headaches produce intense, excruciating pain that can peak in 10 minutes; pain is always unilateral and often associated with tearing and rhinorrhea on the ipsilateral side
        - Can be short lived - average about one hour, but can be longer; occur several times a day and around the same time of day for weeks or months, hence their name
        - *Treatment*
            - 6 mg injection of Sumatriptan, which has the fastest onset of action, as early as five minutes, with pain relief within 15 minutes (also available in nasal spray)
            - Zolmitriptan
            - DHE IV
            - Lidocaine (4%) nose drops
            - Oxygen; 7L/min for up to 10 minutes
            - Nursing: teach correct and timely use of medications
- Pain associated with chronic daily headache (CDH) or recurrent headache related to overuse of medications (analgesic rebound headache) and for treatment of severe cases requiring inpatient detoxification
    o Chronic daily headache: the patient has a headache (not related to a secondary cause) at least 15 days a month; mild to moderate, but not disabling
    o Analgesic rebound for drug overuse headache: as headache becomes more frequent, patients take medication chronically

- o *Treatment*
    - Use of short course of oral steroids to break headache cycle
    - Valproate sodium IV may rapidly break the cycle
    - Inform patient that medication for acute treatment should not be used more than two to three days out of seven (Bader & Littlejohns, 2004).

Prevention

- Avoidance of triggers
- Lifestyle modification
- Hormonal balance
- Pharmacological prophylaxis (Bader & Littlejohns, 2004)

Brain Tumors

What is the clinical presentation of a person with a migraine? What about a brain tumor? What classifications are there?

A brain tumor is an abnormal growth of tissue in the brain. The tumor can either originate in the brain itself (primary brain tumor) or come from another part of the body and travel to the brain (metastatic or secondary brain tumor). Brain tumors may be classified as either benign (non-cancerous) or malignant (cancerous), depending on their behavior (Ohio State University Medical Center, 2013).

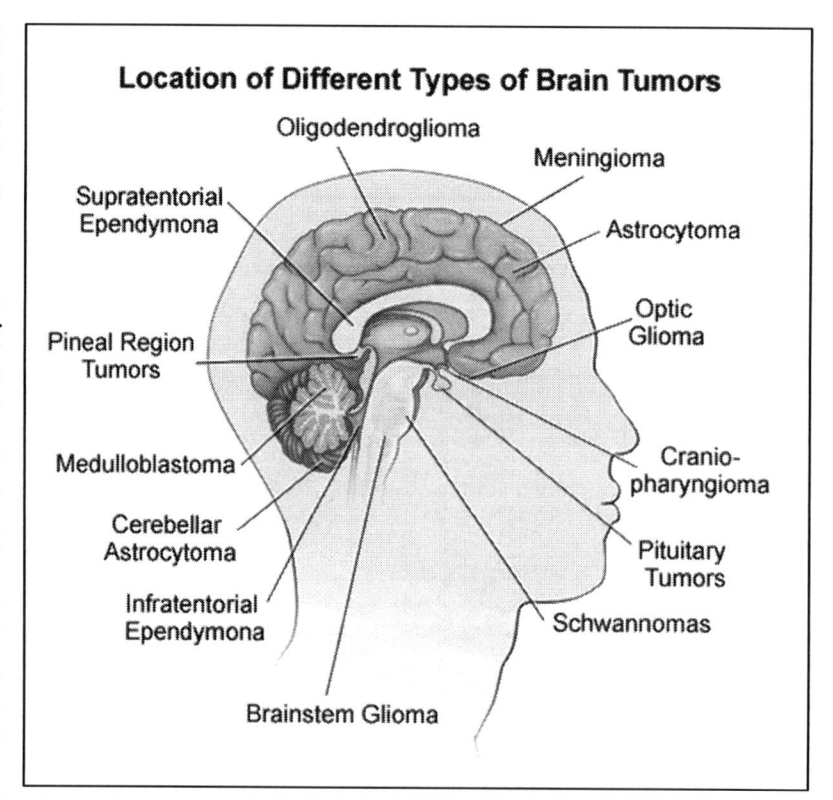

Location of Different Types of Brain Tumors: Oligodendroglioma, Meningioma, Supratentorial Ependymona, Astrocytoma, Pineal Region Tumors, Optic Glioma, Medulloblastoma, Cranio-pharyngioma, Cerebellar Astrocytoma, Pituitary Tumors, Infratentorial Ependymona, Schwannomas, Brainstem Glioma

Epidemiology

- The incidence of primary (malignant and benign) brain tumor is 12.8 per 100,000 (36,400 primary brain tumors nationwide).
- 10-15% of cancer patients develop metastases to the brain (Bader & Littlejohns, 2004).

Etiology and Contributing Factors

- From each primary brain tumor, there arise specific cellular structures. The cause of primary brain tumors remains unknown. Some tumors are thought to be caused by genetic factors or familial history.
- Peak incidence of tumors occurs in the fifth to seventh decade of life
- Higher incidence in men than in women
- Metastatic tumors arise from cancers of the lung (35%), breast (20%), skin (10%), kidney (10%), and gastrointestinal tract (5%) (Bader & Littlejohns, 2004).

Classification and Grading of Tumors

Brain tumors can be classified based on tissue of origin, location, and whether they are primary or metastatic.

- *Astrocytic tumors:* Tumors that form in astrocyte cells. Astrocytic cells perform many functions including biochemical support of endothelial cells that form the blood-brain barrier, provision of nutrients to the nervous tissue, maintenance of extracellular ion balance, and a role in the repair and scarring process of the brain and spinal cord following traumatic injuries.
- *Ologodendroglial tumors and mixed gliomas:* Oligoastrocytomas belong to a group of brain tumors called "gliomas." Gliomas are tumors that come from the glial, or supportive, cells of the brain. There are several different types of gliomas. An oligoastrocytoma is a "mixed glioma" tumor, which contains both abnormal oligodendroglioma and astrocytoma cells.
- *Ependymal tumors:* Tumors that form in the ependymal cells, which are a type of neuronal support cell (neuroglia) that forms the epithelial lining of the ventricles (cavities) in the brain and the central canal of the spinal cord.
- *Choroid plexus tumors*
- *Neuroepithelial tumors of uncertain origin:* An usually supratentorial glial-neuronal neoplasm occurring in children and young adults and characterized by a predominantly cortical location and by drug-resistant partial seizures.
- *Neuronal and mixed neuronal-glial tumors:* These rare, benign tumors come from ganglion-type cells, which are groups of nerve cells. These tumors are commonly located in the temporal lobe of the cerebral hemispheres and the third ventricle. They may also occur in the spine. These tumors are small and slow-growing and have distinct margins. Metastasis and malignancy are very rare.
- *Pineal parenchymal tumors:* Tumors originating in the pineal region, the endocrine gland responsible for the synthesis and secretion of melatonin (the hormone that regulates the sleep cycle). Rare, malignant, and most commonly found in children, these account for less than 1% of primary central nervous system tumors.
- *Embryonal tumors:* Embryonal CNS neoplasms arise within the cerebral hemisphere. This rare group of tumors is most common in children and is rare in adults. *Medulloblastomas and PNET tumors* are types of embryonal tumors.

- *Peripheral neuroblastic tumors:* These are derived from immature sympathetic neuroblasts and are diagnosed in the primary sites related to the embryonic distribution of neural crest cells such as adrenal medulla and structures of the sympathetic nervous system in the thorax, abdomen, and pelvic cavity.
- *Tumors of cranial and peripheral nerves:* Most tumors that arise from cranial and peripheral nerves arise from the Schwann cells and may produce neuro-ophthalmologic symptoms.
- *Meningeal tumors:* Diverse set of tumors arising from the meninges, the membranous layers surrounding the central nervous system. They arise from the arachnoid "cap" cells of the arachnoid villi in the meninges. These tumors are usually benign in nature; however, a small percentage is malignant.
- *Tumors of hematopoietic system:* Malignancies of the hematopoietic and lymphoid tissues include the lymphomas, leukemias, myeloproliferative neoplasms, plasma cell dyscrasias, histiocytic tumors, and dendritic cell neoplasms.
- *Germ cell tumors*: A germ cell tumor (GCT) is a neoplasm derived from germ cells. Germ cell tumors can be cancerous or non-cancerous. Germ cells normally occur inside the gonads (ovary and testis). Germ cell tumors that originate outside the gonads may be birth defects resulting from errors during the development of the embryo.
- *Familial tumor syndromes:* The familial brain tumor syndromes are a heterogeneous group of genetic disorders characterized by a combination of systemic manifestations (often dermatologic) and CNS neoplasms. Some of these syndromes include neurofibromatosis types 1 and 2, tuberous sclerosis, von Hippel-Lindau disease, and Li-Fraumeni syndrome.
- *Tumors of the sellar region:* The sellar and parasellar region is an anatomically complex area that represents a critical junction for important contiguous structures. The most frequently involved structures are the brain parenchyma, meninges, the optic pathways and cranial oculomotor nerves (III, IV, VI) and the V1 and V2 branches of the trigeminal nerve, major blood vessels, hypothalamo-pituitary system, tuber cinereum, anterior third ventricle, and bone compartments.
- *Metastatic tumors of the CNS:* A metastatic brain tumor begins as a cancer elsewhere in the body and spreads to the brain. Sometimes, this process results in a single tumor; approximately 10-20% of all brain metastases are single tumors. However, metastasis sometimes causes multiple tumors (Bader & Littlejohns, 2004).

WHO Grading System for Brain Tumors

The World Health Organization (WHO) grading system is contained in the volume *Histological Typing of Tumors of the Central Nervous System*, whose first edition dates back to 1979, the second to 1993, and the most recent one to 2007. The WHO grading system contains four categories of tumors:

- **Grade I** tumors are slow-growing, non-malignant, and associated with long-term survival.
- **Grade II** tumors are relatively slow-growing, but sometimes recur as higher-grade tumors. They can be non-malignant or malignant.
- **Grade III** tumors are malignant and often recur as higher-grade tumors.
- **Grade IV** tumors reproduce rapidly and are very aggressive malignant tumors (Bader & Littlejohns, 2004).

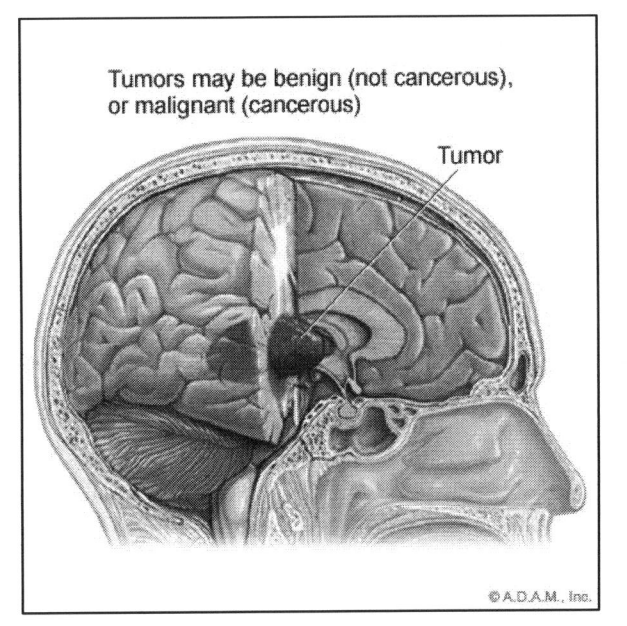

Neuroepithelial Tissue Tumors

Astrocytic tumor (fibrillary, diffuse)
- WHO grade II
- Infiltrating tumor composed primarily of astrocytes

Anaplastic (malignant) Astrocytoma
- WHO grade III
- Peak incidence occurs between 30 and 50 years of age
- Biologically aggressive
  - *Hemispheric*
  - *Diencephalic*
  - *Optic*
  - *Brainstem*
  - *Cerebellar*

Glioblastoma multiforme
- WHO grade IV
- Variants: giant cell glioblastoma, gliosarcoma
- Most rapidly growing, with areas of necrosis; highly infiltrative
- Most frequent and malignant brain tumor in adults; peak incidence occurs between 50 and 70 years of age
- Mean survival is < one year
- Most progress from lower-grade astrocytomas (WHO grade II)
- Found in cerebellar hemisphere
- Causes mass effect on normal structures of the brain

Oligodendroglial Tumors

Oligodendroglioma, low-grade
- WHO grade II

Oligodendroglioma, anaplastic (malignant)
- WHO grade III
- Tumor composed primarily of oligodendroglia cells
- BAD prognosis – high cell density and necrosis
- Structures of Scherer – produced by the affinity of the tumor cells for the cortical gray matter
- Slow growth over a number of years

Ependymal Tumors

Ependymal, low-grade (Ependymoma)
- WHO grade II
- Composed predominantly of ependymal cells
- Tumor typically projects from an ependymal surface
- Slow growth over a number of years
- Prognosis is better in adults than in children
- Intraspinal tumors have a better course than intracranial tumors
- Benign tumor tissue causes complications as it competes for space with CSF

Myxopapillary Ependymoma (WHO grade I)
- Occurs virtually always in the region of the cauda equina
- Originates from the filum terminale or theconus medullaris
- Ependymal cells arranged in a perivascular papillary pattern
- Perivascular and intercellular mucin deposition
- Hemorrhages are frequent

Subependymoma
- Tumor composed of nests of uniform ependymal cells in a stroma of dense acellular fibrillary processes
- Frequently, they present as small asymptomatic nodules
- Others may present as small or large masses projecting into a ventricle, especially the 4th ventricle
- Typically slow-growing

Anaplastic (malignant) Ependymoma (WHO grade III)
- *Schwannoma*
    - Benign neoplasm derived from Schwann cells
    - Occurs on sensory nerves, particularly CN VIII (vestibular)
    - Occurs in adults 20 to 50 years of age
    - Causes compression on affected cranial nerve
- *Neurofibroma*
    - Benign peripheral nerve sheath tumor
    - Multiple lesions are a key feature of neurofibromatosis type I (NF I)

- o Bilateral vestibular Schwannoma (CN VIII) is a key feature of neurofibromatosis type II (NF II) (Bader & Littlejohns, 2004)

Tumors of the Meningeal and Related Tissues

- Slow-growing intracranial neoplasm derived from meningeal cells; well circumscribed; usually not infiltrative; easily excisable
- Arise with bone or pericranial soft tissue
- Common locations: parasagittal, cerebral convexity, sphenoid ridge, sellar, olfactory grove
- Usually occur in adults, more often in women than in men
- Cause compression on brain tissue (Bader & Littlejohns, 2004)

Hematopoietic Tumors

- Primary malignant lymphomas
  - o Cause elevated ICP and brain destruction
- Tumors of blood vessel origin (hemangioblastomas)
  - o Highly vascular tumors; may be a cyst
  - o Usually found in cerebellum, brainstem, or cervical spine
  - o Presents in adults 20 to 40 years of age
  - o Genetically associated with VHL disease
  - o Impedes CSF flow, causing elevated ICP (Bader & Littlejohns, 2004)

Pituitary Tumors

- Neoplasms derived from cells of the anterior pituitary gland, typically solitary tumors
- Benign tumors, but cause endocrine dysfunctions (Cushing's disease), acromegaly, prolactinoma; can compress optic chiasm, distend sella turcica, or encroach upon cavernous sinus

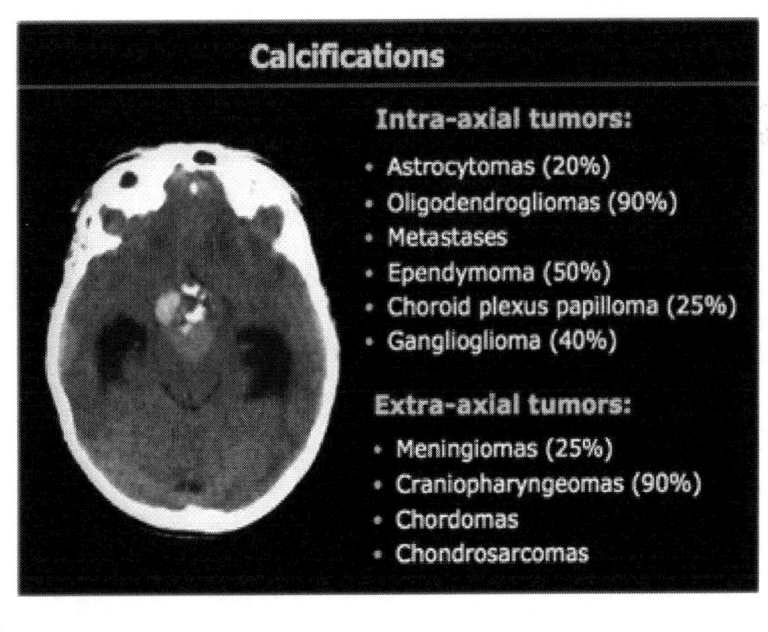

Calcifications

Intra-axial tumors:
- Astrocytomas (20%)
- Oligodendrogliomas (90%)
- Metastases
- Ependymoma (50%)
- Choroid plexus papilloma (25%)
- Ganglioglioma (40%)

Extra-axial tumors:
- Meningiomas (25%)
- Craniopharyngeomas (90%)
- Chordomas
- Chondrosarcomas

- Microadenoma <1cm; macroadenoma >1cm
- 10-20% of all intracranial neoplasms found in the pituitary region
- Higher incidence in adults 20 to 50 years of age; found in women more than in men; occasionally found in children

Craniopharyngioma

- Tumor is considered by some people to originate from remnants of the craniopharyngeal duct (Rathke's pouch)
- Calcified cystic suprasella mass filled with a dark brown fluid
- Usually occurs in first two decades of life
- Common features: calcification, wet keratin, ossification, and inflammatory reaction

Cerebellar and Brainstem Tumors

- Most common infratentorial tumors; typically occur between birth and 20 years of age; hemangioblastoma, brainstem glioma, cavernous hemangioma, metastasis
- Features: some tumor types can seed into ventricles or craniospinal axis
- Typically cause cerebellar signs (ataxia, incoordination, CSF obstruction, and brainstem compression) (Bader & Littlejohns, 2004)

Metastatic Tumors

- Most common primary sites: lung (35%), breast (20%), skin (10%), kidney (10%), gastrointestinal tract (5%)
- Typical features: spherical, contrast-enhancing with a necrotic center and peritumoral edema; usually occur in gray matter near major arteries, especially in the middle cerebral artery; can present with multiple lesions (melanomas) or solitary lesion (kidney, GI tract)
- Surgical resection as an option depends on multiple factors including radio sensitivity of the brain lesion, type of tumor, location, number of brain lesions, estimated life expectancy, and presence or absence of other systemic metastases (Bader & Littlejohns, 2004).

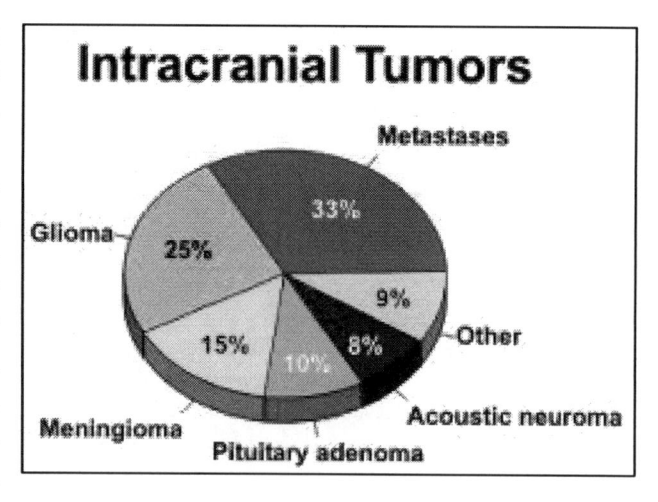

Tumors of the Pineal Region

Germinoma

- Most frequent tumor in the pineal region
- Biphasic
- Indistinguishable from testicular seminoma and the ovarian dysgerminoma

- Radio sensitive
- Other germ cell tumors in the pineal region: embryonal carcinoma, yolk sac tumor, choriocarcinoma, and teratoma

Pineocytoma (WHO grade III)

- Uncommon tumor composed of pineal cells
- Polar processes radiate towards the vascular stroma with club-like expansions at their tips
- Malignant tumor
- Behaves as benign when it exhibits neuronal differentiation

Pineoblastoma (WHO grade IV)

- Rare, highly cellular pineal tumor
- Consists of small, poorly differentiated cells (PNET cells)
- Always a malignant tumor

Astrocytic Tumors

- Benign and malignant astrocytic tumors may occur in the pineal gland

Hemangioblastoma

- Cystic, capillary-rich neoplasm containing variably lipidized stromal cells
- Occurs either sporadically (70%) or in association with the von Hippel-Lindau disease (30%)
- Prototypic hemangioblastoma - cystic cerebellar mass with a contrast-enhancing mural nodule

Primary Central Nervous System Lymphoma

- Deep-seated tumors
- Solitary in healthy people
- Multiple in immunocompromised patients
- Most are B-cell lymphomas
- Being centered around arteries and angioinvasion are characteristic (Bader & Littlejohns, 2004)

Assessment

- Headache is seen in about 50% of patients
  - Dull, vague ache; more typically, a headache that is progressive in severity, worse in the morning, or occurs when they are recumbent
  - If HA is associated with projectile vomiting, this suggests increased ICP and must be handled quickly

- Mental status changes including confusion, short-term memory loss, personality changes, mood swings, lethargy, or depression
- Visual symptoms: blurring, diplopia, or decreased peripheral vision
- Seizures: focal or generalized; often a good prognostic factor because patients experiencing seizures may have their tumors discovered more quickly
- Objective-focal neurological deficits
- Ataxia, gait disturbance
- Hemisensory or motor deficit, asymmetrical reflexes (Bader & Littlejohns, 2004)

Diagnosis

- Labs
    - No serum tumor markers available for primary brain tumors
    - Pituitary tumors may secrete prolactin, corticotropin, and/or growth hormone
- EEG: used to document seizure focus and focal slowing of brain waves
- CT scan: helpful in evaluating bony lesions of the skull or spine, calcifications, or hemorrhage, but can miss smaller parenchymal lesions, particularly in posterior fossa
- MRI: shows structure in three planes with or without gadolinium; the examination of choice for primary and metastatic brain tumors; *low-grade tumors do not enhance whereas higher-grade tumors enhance due to greater disruption of the blood-brain barrier (BBB)*
- MRA: non-invasive method of visualizing vascular structures
- Functional MRI: detects physiological changes during physical and cognitive activity
- Magnetic resonance spectroscopy: measures level of metabolites to help differentiate necrosis from scarring from malignancy
- Thallium 201 single photon emission CT: can help differentiate tumor versus radiation necrosis
- Position emission tomography scan: measures tissue metabolism
- Lumbar puncture: for suspicion of leptomeningeal involvement or in evaluation of medulloblastoma or lymphoma
- CSF flow scan: evaluates CSF flow abnormalities, particularly in patients with leptomeningeal disease or tumors within the ventricular system
- Pathology: necessary for accurate diagnosis and treatment decisions; tissue may be obtained by biopsy or craniotomy
- Cellular proliferation measures: higher degree of proliferation correlates with higher-grade, more aggressive tumor; less favorable prognosis
- Tumor typing: can help individualize treatment plans (Bader & Littlejohns, 2004)

Prognosis

- Currently, it is a product of tumor histology, extent of surgical resection, clinical performance status, and age (Bader & Littlejohns, 2004).

Treatment

- Treatment is multidisciplinary including surgery, radiation, and/or chemotherapy
- Primary tumors - craniotomy for maximum resection, if possible
- Biopsy - small sample of tumor removed to obtain pathological diagnosis
- Metastatic tumors - one or more lesions may be resected
- Lymphomas - require only a biopsy and are not resected, thus chemo/radiation therapy is treatment choice
- Pituitary tumors - transphenoidal approach is often employed
- MRI performed within 24 to 72 hours post-op
- Radiation therapy
    - Ionizing radiation - to damage cellular DNA
    - Cells most sensitive to radiation are those that are rapidly dividing, that are in a mitotic phase, or that are immature
    - Brachytherapy - radioactive isotopes are placed in the tumor or resection cavity to provide high dose in a localized area
- Chemotherapy interventions - work at the cellular level to slow or prevent the proliferation of abnormal cell
- Steroid therapy (oral or IV) - to reduce cerebral edema
    - Monitor for side effects (thrush, immunosuppression)
- Seizure prevention
- Pain management (*brain parenchyma does not contain pain receptors*) (Bader & Littlejohns, 2004)

Nursing Interventions

- Critical care, acute care, perioperative period: monitor ICP and vitals, and make frequent neuro checks
- Acute nursing interventions during radiation - monitor skin integrity and implement measures to protect and restore if altered; educate on skin care, and make referrals for wigs or hats; monitor for hearing loss and fatigue, and provide fatigue management strategies
- Acute and chronic nursing interventions for patients undergoing chemotherapy - be reassuring; help patient maintain a positive attitude; teach patient about side effects of treatment; administer antiemetics; monitor CBC with differential
- *General guidelines for treatment with chemotherapy - ANC >1500 (absolute neutrophil count); hemoglobin >10.0; platelets >100,000*
- Council patients on nutrition, mouth care, and rest
- Treat side effects from chemotherapy
    - Altered taste sensation (dysgeusia), which can impact nutrition
    - Metallic taste in mouth - most prominent with meat consumption; zinc may help
    - Refer to nutritionist who specializes in working with chemotherapy patients
    - Assess for anorexia, cachexia, weight loss, and muscle wasting
    - Antiemetic given routinely to prevent nausea
    - Add protein to diet (milk, whey protein)

- o Encourage patient to eat small, frequent meals
- Administer antidepressants; may improve function as well as mood
  - o Potential for dysphoria or depression
- Encourage birth control in females of childbearing age
  - o Patients may need reproductive counseling *before* treatment
- Refer to occupational therapy and cognitive rehabilitation
- Administer steroids as prescribed and monitor for side effects
- Refer to social work, palliative care, or hospice services
- Patient should be encouraged to complete advanced directives
- Refer to pastoral care/spiritual support
- Treat anemia, if indicated
  - o Encourage rest and activity, as tolerated
- Encourage support groups and respite services for patient and family
- Give ongoing teaching throughout the continuum
- Give honest, correct information while maintaining hope (Bader & Littlejohns, 2004)

Spinal Cord Tumors

- Spinal cord tumors usually occur between 20 and 60 years of age
- 60% of tumors are benign in adults; children have a higher incidence of gliomas and sarcoma tumors

Epidemiology

- One tenth as common as brain tumors; about 1,500 cases per year
- In adults, 60% are benign
- Children have a higher incidence of gliomas and sarcomas
- Distribution of vertebral column correlates with the amount of cord tissue in each area:
  - o Thoracic 50%
  - o Lumbar 25%
  - o Cervical 20%
  - o Cauda equina 5%
- Approximately 5% of cancer patients will have a spinal cord metastasis from systemic cancer of the breast, lung, or prostate (Bader & Littlejohns, 2004).

Etiology

- Cause unknown
- Genetic
- Von Recklinghausen disease (neurofibromatosis)

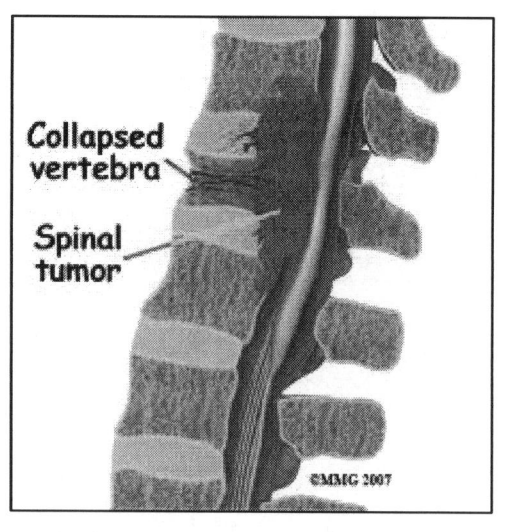

- Primary (e.g. astrocytoma, ependymoma, meningioma)

Metastatic

- Extradural
- Primary, usually lung, breast, or prostate
- In 10% of patients, initial symptom of disease is spinal cord metastasis
- 17-30% of patients have two or more cord lesions
- Symptoms
    - Pain - localized with percussion of vertebral column
    - Weakness of extremities
    - Bowel and bladder problems

Neurofibroma

- Von Recklinghausen disease
- Benign tumor
- Usually occurs in the thoracic spine
- May occur in multiple lesions
- Initial symptom: nerve root compression
- Treatment: surgical resection

Classification of Tumor Type

Spinal cord tumors can occur within or adjacent to the spinal cord. They are considered to be intra-axial in location and can be either primary or metastatic. Primary spinal cord tumors account for 2-4% of all primary central nervous system tumors, one-third of which are located in the intramedullary compartment. Spinal cord tumors can be classified according to their anatomic location:

- ***Intramedullary*** - Intramedullary tumors arise within the spinal cord itself. Most primary intramedullary tumors are either ependymomas or astrocytomas.
- ***Intradural-extramedullary*** - Tumors arising within the dura, but outside the actual spinal cord, are termed intradural-extramedullary. The most common tumors in this group are Schwannoma, meningiomas, and nerve sheath tumors.
- ***Extradural*** - Extradural tumors are usually metastatic and most often arise in the vertebral bodies. Metastatic lesions can cause spinal cord compression either by epidural growth that results in extrinsic spinal cord or cauda equina compression or less frequently by intradural invasion that can also develop into surrounding bones or vertebral bodies (Bader & Littlejohns, 2004; Welch, Schiff, & Gerszten, 2013).

Pathophysiology

- ***Cord compression***
    - Traction on or irritation of spinal nerve roots
    - Spinal cord displacement

- o Altered blood supply - risk for infarct
- o Spinal cord responds to pressure from edema, which can ascend and cause neurological deficits at a higher cord segment
- o Obstruction of CSF flow
- *Direct pressure on spinal cord*
  - o Interferes with spinal nerve root and cord conduction
  - o Impairs blood flow to spinal veins below level of pressure and produces edema
- *Invasion of spinal cord*
  - o Destroys or invades spinal cord substance itself
  - o Destroys spinal cord parenchyma
- *Vertebral bony metastasis*
  - o Tumor cells are disseminated through circulatory system
  - o Destruction of cortical bone by tumor
  - o Vertebral body collapse - risk for fracture and paralysis (Bader & Littlejohns, 2004)
- *Tumor progression*
  - o Benign
    - Slow-growing
    - Few neurological signs
  - o Malignant
    - Fast-growing
    - Acute due to hemorrhage into cord
    - Acute flaccid paresis from lesion downward (Bader & Littlejohns, 2004)

Assessment

- Subjective - pain, weakness, bowel and bladder dysfunction, numbness, tingling
- Objective - specific to tumor type
  - o *Extradural*
    - *Metastatic*
      - Primary, usually in lung, breast, or prostate
      - May have multiple lesions
      - Symptoms include pain on percussion of vertebral column, weakness of extremities, and bowel and bladder problems
    - *Extramedullary/intradural*
      - Schwannoma (most common)
        - Benign tumor
        - Usually in thoracic spine
        - Dumbbell or hourglass configuration
        - Initial symptom: nerve root compression
        - Treatment: surgical excision
      - Neurofibroma (Von Recklinghausen disease/neurofibromatosis)
        - Benign tumor
        - Usually in thoracic spine
        - May occur in multiple locations

- Initial symptom: nerve root compression
- Treatment: surgical resection
- Meningioma
  - Benign
  - 60% occurrence in thoracic spine
  - Women 40 to 60 years of age
  - Can be highly vascular
  - Occurs posterolateral to spinal cord and dural base
  - Symptoms include:
    - Long tract signs: spasticity, hyperreflexia, and abnormal reflexes such as Babinski or Hoffman's sign
    - Brown Sequard syndrome: by loss of motor function (example: hemiparaplegia), loss of vibration sense and fine touch, loss of proprioception (position sense), loss of two-point discrimination, and signs of weakness on the ipsilateral (same side) of the spinal injury (Bader & Littlejohns, 2004)
- *Intramedullary/intradural*
  - *Astrocytoma*
    - Occurs within the spinal substance
    - Well differentiated; may become malignant
    - Occurs more in males
    - Half accompanied by cystic component
    - Symptoms:
      - Long tract signs
      - Unilateral or bilateral paresis
      - Sensory level
      - Bowel and bladder problems
    - Rapid growth
    - Treatment:
      - Surgical aspiration of cystic component and bulk resection
      - Radiation therapy
    - Prognosis based on level of malignancy (Bader & Littlejohns, 2004)
  - *Ependymoma*
    - Accounts for 10% of all cord tumors
    - Half occur in cauda equina including lumbar, sacral, conus medullaris, and filum terminale
    - Most are intramedullary
    - Rarely malignant; if it is, it can spread rapidly through spinal and cranial areas
    - Symptoms:
      - Initially, pain or weakness of extremity
      - Local vertebral pain
      - Radicular pain
      - Bladder symptoms
    - Treatment:
      - Surgical resection possible

- If resection not possible, radiation and possibly chemotherapy (Bader & Littlejohns, 2004)
  - *Hemangioblastoma*
    - Malignant, but not fatal
    - Associated with VHL disease
    - Slow-growing
    - Tumor associated with syringomyelia and cystic component
    - Treatment:
      - Surgical resection possible
      - Radiation to retard growth (Bader & Littlejohns, 2004)
  - *Epidermoids, dermoids*
    - Congenital tumors
    - Benign, slow-growing
    - Avascular, capsulated
    - Occur in the lumbar area (Bader & Littlejohns, 2004)
  - *Occur in the lumbar region*
    - Associated with spina bifida
    - Associated with dermal sinus tract
    - Easily resectable; can recur after subtotal resection (Bader & Littlejohns, 2004)

Patient Problems/Interventions

Acute neurological impairment due to spinal cord tumor
- Sudden and progressive motor impairment
- Sudden and progressive sensory impairment
- Acute manifestation due to hemorrhage into tumor or spinal cord (Bader & Littlejohns, 2004)

Pain due to cord compression
- Pain increase in supine position; decreases when sitting upright; exact opposite of disk disease
- Pain with vertebral palpation (Bader & Littlejohns, 2004)

Altered elimination: bowel and bladder dysfunctions
- Paralytic ileus and constipation
- Frequent urinary tract infections
- Urinary retention
- Continuous dribble of urine (Bader & Littlejohns, 2004)

Altered skin integrity
- Altered sensation or motor function below level of lesion
- Altered healing with use of corticosteroids and administration of radiation (Bader & Littlejohns, 2004)

Interventions
- Curative vs. palliative
  - Benign tumor: curative, if totally resectable
  - Metastatic tumor: palliative for symptom and pain management

- o Metastatic tumor with aggressive systemic disease: radiation only for palliation
- Medications
  - o High-dose steroids (corticosteroids)
  - o Opioids: sustained release and transdermal
  - o Intrathecal opioids: may not be appropriate with presence of spinal cord tumor or block
  - o Anticonvulsants for neuropathic pain due to nerve injury
  - o Antidepressants for neuropathic pain
  - o Stool softeners or suppositories for bowel stimulation
  - o Antibiotics for UTIs
- Metastatic lesions: appropriate chemotherapy and endocrine therapy for breast or prostate primary tumors
- Surgical intervention:
  - o Complete or partial resection of tumor and decompression of bony structures
  - o Implantable pump for pain management
- Radiation therapy
  - o Spinal cord can tolerate 4000 to 5000 rads over 5 weeks; 3000 rads may be used for palliative radiation
  - o Pain relief is delayed 2 to 6 weeks
  - o Side effects: radiation-induced myelopathy; chronic progressive sensory impairment at level of cord radiated; loss of sensation; loss of bowel and bladder control
- Interventional radiology
  - o Percutaneous vertebroplasty
    - A needle is placed fluroscopically into collapsed vertebral body and filled with polymethylmethacrylate (bone cement) to fill up space
    - Provides support and stabilization
    - Cement releases heat, which destroys nerve endings, which decreases pain
    - Immediate improvement of pain
    - Most patients experience full benefit after 6 months
- Nursing interventions
  - o Preoperative and post-operative neurological assessment
  - o Family and patient education
  - o Initiation of physical therapy and occupational therapy
  - o Pain assessment and documentation of pain scale
  - o Around-the-clock dosing, not as needed
  - o Patient and family education about pain management
  - o Proper positioning for comfort and body mechanics
  - o Monitor I/O
  - o Monitor bowel sounds
  - o Monitor daily bowel and bladder habits - implement toilet training, if necessary
  - o Promote peaceful environment to promote rest and relaxation
  - o Bladder scans as needed - insert Foley catheter only if necessary

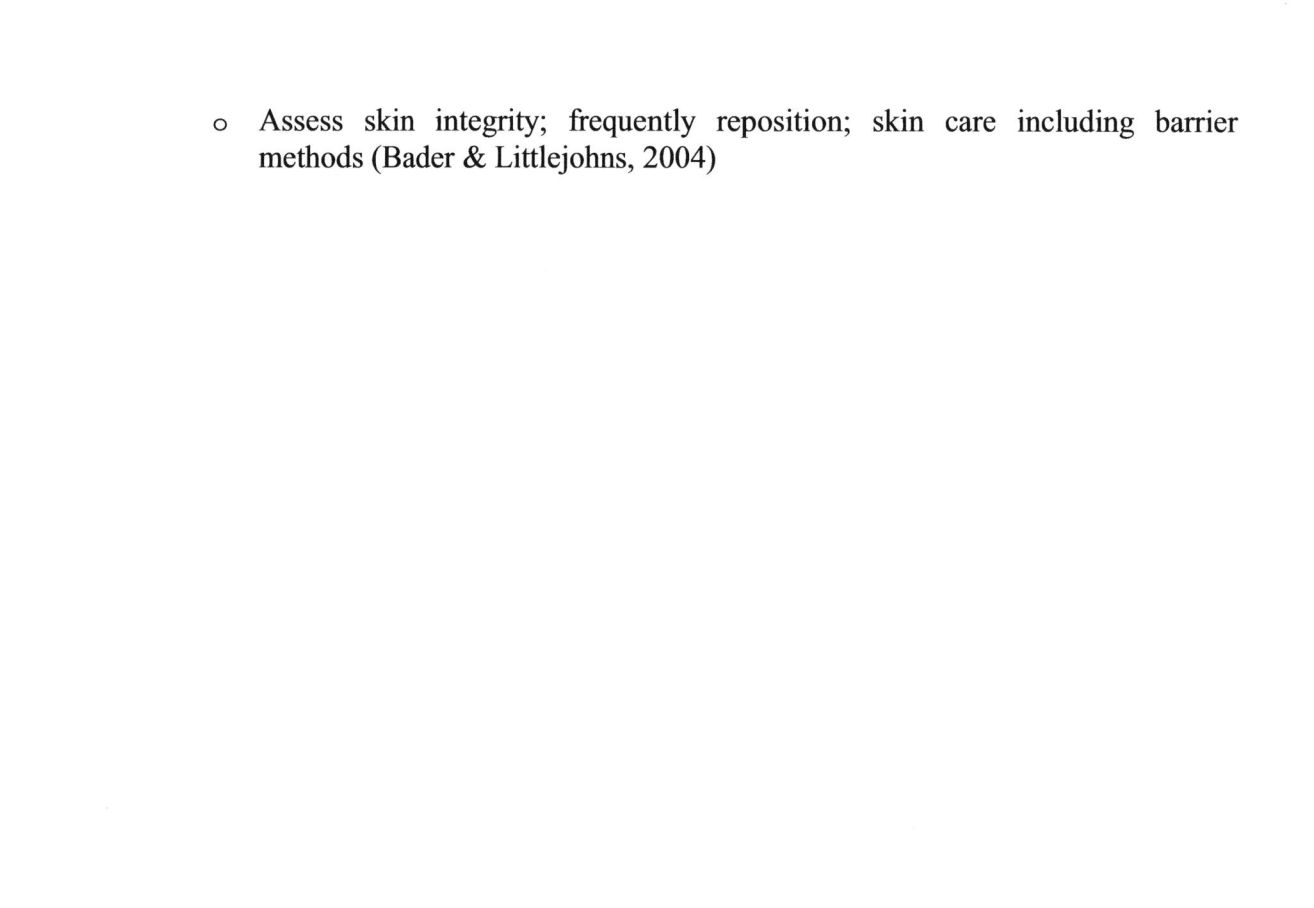

- Assess skin integrity; frequently reposition; skin care including barrier methods (Bader & Littlejohns, 2004)

Chapter 4: Immune and Infectious Disorders of the Neurological System

Abscesses (Intracranial)

A brain abscess is encapsulated or free pus in the brain tissue, usually secondary to an infection elsewhere in the body (Bader & Littlejohns, 2004).

Epidemiology

- Brain abscesses account for nearly 1% of the space-occupying brain lesions in the U.S.
- Incidences of such infections are more prevalent in underdeveloped countries.
- Increased opportunistic infections in immunocompromised hosts are contributing to the incidence of abscesses (Bader & Littlejohns, 2004).

Etiology and Contributing Factors

- 40% are an extension of the middle ear, mastoid, and paranasal sinuses
- Infections occur through osteomyelitis of the bone or travel along the veins
- Such extensions are likely to be a single abscess located in the frontal and temporal lobes
- 30% are a result of metastasis from elsewhere in the body (pulmonary infections, acute bacterial endocarditis, or infection associated with congenital heart defects)
- Multiple abscesses may be present and can be difficult to differentiate from metastatic lesions.
- Organisms are carried by the bloodstream and are held within the distribution of the middle cerebral artery.
- 10% are the result of penetrating trauma, skull fracture, and neurosurgical procedure
- 20% are of unknown etiology
- More common in males, particularly in the first 20 years of life
- Immunocompromised patients are at highest risk for developing (Bader & Littlejohns, 2004)

Pathophysiology

- Abscesses develop in four stages:
    o Cerebritis with necrotic center surrounded by an inflammatory response
    o Pus formation with proliferation of inflammatory cells, macrophages, and increased edema
    o Capsule formation from fibroblasts, which creates a "ring" or "halo;" this limits the spread of infection and prevents destruction of brain parenchyma
    o Mature abscess with a necrotic center, a zone of inflammatory cells, a capsule, and edema surrounding the capsule

- The organism is directly related to the site of origin
  - Anaerobic organisms, especially *streptococci* from ear and dental infections
  - *Staphylococcus aureus* from sinus infections
  - Pulmonary infections
  - Fungal infections in immunocompromised patients
    - Parasitic infections are also present in patients with HIV (Bader & Littlejohns, 2004)

Prevention

- Early recognition and appropriate treatment of existing infections can reduce the incidence of brain abscesses (Bader & Littlejohns, 2004)

Assessment

- Subjective - progressive headache
- Objective data
  - Similar to those of a tumor or space-occupying lesion; develop rapidly over two weeks
  - History of a primary infection
  - Primary symptoms include fever, nausea and vomiting, altered LOC, focal neurological deficits, and seizures
- Diagnostics
  - Laboratory studies - show mild WBC count increase and elevated erythrocyte sedimentation rate
  - Lumbar puncture: risky procedure due to the intracranial mass, elevated opening pressure, and mild increase in protein level
  - Radiography of chest, skull, and sinuses can identify primary infection site.
  - CT: can facilitate both early diagnosis and staging of the abscess; metastatic infections produce multiple lesions
  - MRI: similar to CT scan; in addition, able to differentiate liquid necrosis from edema (Bader & Littlejohns, 2004)

Treatment

- Antibiotic therapy
  - Directed to the specific organism based on culture and sensitivity testing
  - Before culture is obtained, the choice is to treat for the organism most encountered
  - Antibiotics alone may manage small abscesses (< 2 cm)
  - Long-term therapy is given for six weeks
- Surgical intervention
  - Epidural abscesses > 2.5 cm should be treated surgically
  - Approach determined by age and neurological status, location of lesion, and number of lesions

- o Aspiration via burr hole can provide decompression and culture specimen
- o Craniotomy is used to remove abscess and contaminated bone or material; not preferred for deep abscesses
- Nursing interventions
  - o Same care as provided with bacterial meningitis
  - o Home healthcare for long-term antibiotic therapy (Bader & Littlejohns, 2004)

Intracranial Epidural Abscesses

An epidural abscess develops between the skull and dura mater and is associated with an overlying osteomyelitis (Bader & Littlejohns, 2004).

Epidemiology

- Cranial epidural abscesses are rare; 1.8% occur status post clean craniotomy
- Incidence is higher after craniofacial surgery (Bader & Littlejohns, 2004)

Etiology and Contributing Factors

- Trauma, surgery, paranasal sinusitis, and mastoiditis are highly contributory
- Often associated with bacteremia, drug use, and immunocompromised conditions (Bader & Littlejohns, 2004)

Pathophysiology

- Pus and granulation material accrue on the outer surface of the dura
- *S. aureus* is most common organism identified (Bader & Littlejohns, 2004)

Prevention

- Early recognition and appropriate treatment of existing infections can reduce the incidence of cranial epidural abscesses (Bader & Littlejohns, 2004)

Assessment

- Subjective - mild frontal headache from sinuses or ear
- Objective - purulent drainage from the ears, low-grade fever, moderate nuchal rigidity
- Diagnosis - lumbar puncture, CT scan, MRI (Bader & Littlejohns, 2004)

Treatment

- Antibiotics
- Supportive therapy
- Surgical - aspiration via burr hole, insertion of subdural drains, cranioplasty (Bader & Littlejohns, 2004)

Spinal Epidural Abscess

A spinal epidural abscess is an accumulation of purulent fluid above the dura surrounding the spinal cord (Bader & Littlejohns, 2004).

Epidemiology

- Spinal epidural abscesses are rare, but can result in permanent paralysis

Etiology

- 50% of spinal epidural abscesses represent a metastases from other sites such as skin infection, pharyngitis, dental abscess, pelvic inflammatory disease, middle ear infection, sinusitis, and pulmonary infection
- Other risks: spinal surgery, epidural catheters, or injections; history of bacteremia, and drug or alcohol abuse; immunocompromised condition
- Parenteral injections are associated with infections in the cervical region (Bader & Littlejohns, 2004).

Pathophysiology

- Purulent material and granulation tissue cover the spinal dura and may extend over several segments
- Abscess can be associated with vertebral osteomyelitis
- *S. aureus* is most common organism
- Tuberculosis is common with chronic infections of the epidural space
- Vascular occlusions contribute to neurological deficits (Bader & Littlejohns, 2004)

Assessment

- Subjective data
    - Early symptoms are aching in the spinal area with local tenderness
    - With progression, the back pain becomes (and the patient complains of) radicular pain (specific to the site of the abscess)
- Objective data
    - Fever, malaise, and chills
    - Sensory loss with or without motor deficits
    - Neurological deficits may begin with the loss of bowel and bladder function and progress to paraplegia or quadriplegia
- Diagnostics
    - Lumbar puncture: CSF studies show elevated lymphocytes and protein levels
    - CT: reveals bone destruction, extradural, and mass effect
    - MRI: preferred imaging technique for inflammation and lesions of the spinal cord

- o Myelogram: reveals extradural compression and blockage of the spinal canal (Bader & Littlejohns, 2004)

Treatment

- Antibiotic therapy: initiated on diagnosis and modified when organism is identified
- Surgical: extensive decompression laminectomy with evacuation of the purulent liquid and granulation tissue should be performed as soon as possible
- Nursing interventions: same as with bacterial meningitis (Bader & Littlejohns, 2004)

Outcomes

- 50% recover
- 25% have a significant neurological deficit
- 10% are paralyzed
- Mortality rate is 14-30% (Bader & Littlejohns, 2004)

Subdural Empyema

A subdural empyema is a collection of purulent fluid between the inner surface of the dura mater and outer surface of the arachnoid. An empyema is an infection in a pre-existing space. A subdural empyema is a life-threatening infection and must be treated immediately with surgery because increased ICP can lead to cerebral herniation and death (Bader & Littlejohns, 2004).

Epidemiology

- Condition is infrequent and more common in males (Bader & Littlejohns, 2004)

Etiology

- Infection of the paranasal sinuses is most common cause
- Usually aerobic or anaerobic streptococci, Bacteroides species, or *S. aureus* (Bader & Littlejohns, 2004)

Pathophysiology

- The infection often begins in the frontal lobe or ethmoid sinuses and spreads by direct extension through the bone and dura; it is rarely metastatic.
- The amount of subdural pus ranges from a few milliliters to 200 ml, depressing the cerebral cortex and infiltrating the arachnoid; Thrombi develop in the cerebral veins (Bader & Littlejohns, 2004).

Prevention

- Early recognition and appropriate treatment of existing infections can reduce the incidence of subdural empyemas (Bader & Littlejohns, 2004).

Assessment

- Subjective data - headache, pain over the brow, and malaise; other symptoms dependent upon organism involved (Bader & Littlejohns, 2004)
- Objective data
    - History of chronic sinusitis or mastoiditis
    - Fever
    - Stiff neck
    - Focal neurological signs of hemiplegia, sensory loss, and aphasia
    - Seizures
    - Stupor by coma
- Diagnostics
    - Lumbar puncture: risky to perform due to the intracranial mass; elevated opening pressure with a mild increase in protein level
    - CT: may not reveal the early changes associated with subdural empyema
    - MRI: preferred diagnostic test; shows enhancement of the meninges and pus collection
    - Skull and sinus radiographs: to evaluate paranasal sinus infections and mastoiditis (Bader & Littlejohns, 2004)

Treatment

- Antibiotic therapy: initial treatment is penicillin with a third-generation cephalosporin and metronidazole (Flagyl)
- Surgical
    - Surgical emergency: burr holes are drilled to drain subdural empyemas
    - Craniotomy may be required depending on location
    - Nursing: same as with bacterial meningitis

Amyotrophic Lateral Sclerosis

Amyotrophic lateral sclerosis (ALS) is a motor neuronal disease that affects cells in the brain and spinal cord that control voluntary muscle movement. ALS is also known as Lou Gehrig's disease (Bader & Littlejohns, 2004).

Motor Neuron Variants

- Primary lateral sclerosis (PLS)
    - Upper motor neuron (UMN)
    - Prognosis: survival in the decades; progressive decline

- Progressive bulbar palsy (PBP)
    - UMN, lower motor neuron (LMN), or both
    - Bulbar palsy symptoms
        - Dysphagia, difficulty chewing, nasal regurgitation, slurring of speech, choking on liquids, dysphonia (defective use of the voice), dysarthria (difficulty in articulating words), and dysphasia
    - Prognosis: poor due to nutritional and respiratory compromise
- Progressive muscular atrophy (PMA)
    - LMN only
    - Prognosis: similar to that of ALS (Bader & Littlejohns, 2004)
- Asymmetric distal weakness is greater than proximal weakness
    - Both UMN and LMN symptoms
    - Presentation predominance
        - 36% of symptoms in lower extremities
        - 32% of symptoms in upper extremities
        - Bulbar symptoms in 25%
        - Thoracic symptoms (respiratory, truncal) in 7%

Epidemiology

- Sporadic; unknown cause
- Genetic
    - 20% of all cases are familial
    - Chromosomal defects (Bader & Littlejohns, 2004)

Classification El Escorial Criteria

- Demoted by regions and presence of UMN and LMN signs
    - Regions consist of brainstem, cervical, thoracic, and lumbosacral
- Categories
    - Possible UMN and LMN signs in one region
    - Possible UMN and LMN signs in two regions
    - Definite UMN and LMN signs in three regions (Bader & Littlejohns, 2004)

What is ALS?

ALS (Amyotrophic Lateral Sclerosis), also known as Lou Gehrig's disease, is a fatal disease of the nervous system, characterized by progressive muscle weakness resulting in paralysis.

What are motor neurons?

Motor neurons are nerve cells in the brain and spinal cord that attach to muscles and control voluntary movement.

How does ALS progress?

When motor neurons gradually degenerate and die, the muscles no longer receive nerve impulses. As a result of the nerve death, the muscles shrink and waste away.

A closer look at a healthy nervous system

Nervous system

The basic unit of the nervous system is a highly specialized cell, known as a neuron. Its main purpose is to transport messages from one part of the body to another in the form of nerve impulses.

Motor neuron

A motor neuron is made up of three main functional parts.
- **Cell body:** biosynthetic center of the cell
- **Axon:** responsible for sending messages
- **Dendrites:** responsible for receiving messages

Nerve impulse

A nerve impulse is transmitted when the terminal fibers of one neuron's axon release chemicals called neurotransmitters that attach to dendrites of the receptor neurons.

A possible cause of ALS: Too much glutamate

Scientists aren't sure what causes ALS, but glutamate poisoning is a popular theory. Glutamate is an amino acid that acts as a neurotransmitter, allowing motor neurons to "talk" to one another. After transmitting a message, glutamate is supposed to be vacuumed up by a cell membrane protein. But researchers at Johns Hopkins University in Baltimore suggest people with ALS don't have enough of that protein. Over time, glutamate clogs the synaptic cleft, the space between nerve endings, and chokes motor neurons to death. The drug Rilutek slows the body's production of glutamate and keeps ALS patients alive for an extra two to three months.

Dulcie Teasdale/Huntsville Times

106

Pathophysiology

- *Theoretical models*
    - Excitotoxicity: glutamate defect in metabolism, transport, and/or storage
    - Oxidative stress: excess free radicals
    - Autoimmune
        - Antibodies to calcium channels
        - Activated T lymphocytes
        - Monoclonal paraproteinemia
    - Cytoskeletal
        - Neurofilament abnormalities: abnormal accumulation and damage to structure (Bader & Littlejohns, 2004)

Assessment

- Subjective
    - Progressive weakness over weeks to months
    - No sensory abnormalities
    - Muscle atrophy
- Objective
    - Decrease or absence of muscle strength
    - Hyperreflexia, fasciculations
    - Spasticity may or may not be present
- Diagnostics
    - Labs: CK normal or slightly elevated
    - Electrophysiology
        - EMG
            - Denervation
            - Fibrillations, positive sharp waves, fasciculations, large motor units
            - Abnormal findings should be in several regions
        - NCV: normal
        - Motor unit number estimate (MUNE): quantifies number of surviving motor units; sensitive indicator of disease progression
    - Muscle biopsy
        - Numerous small regions grouped with regular atrophic muscle fibers
        - Little fiber type grouping; fiber size variations (Bader & Littlejohns, 2004)

Potential Problems/Interventions

- Risk for self-care deficits, impaired respiratory function, impaired swallowing, aspiration, malnutrition, impaired communication, anxiety, and immobility (Bader & Littlejohns, 2004)
- Medical interventions
    - Pulmonology consult
    - Non-invasive ventilation-Bipap (positive pressure), Cuirass, body wrap, pneumobelt

- Invasive ventilation - tracheostomy and mechanical ventilator
- Cough-assist devices
- Portable suction
- Anticholinergics
- Feeding gastrostomy tube
- NSAIDs (strong caution using narcotics in these patients because of CO2 narcosis)
- Amitriptyline (Elavil) and Neurodex for anxiety
- Nursing interventions
  - Auscultate lung sounds
  - Manage changes in status, per protocols
  - Encourage energy conservation
  - Encourage expression of feelings about disease progression
  - Encourage use of ventilator support (non-invasive/invasive)
  - Help patient use critical-decision thinking when contemplating invasive ventilator support
  - Elevate head of bed with upper extremities supported to improve ventilation
  - Perform bedside swallow evaluation
  - Weigh
  - Notify speech therapist of findings
  - Seek nutritionist for support
  - Help patient use critical-decision thinking when considering artificial feeding
  - Encourage reflective activities
  - Explain advanced directives and assist in paperwork completion
  - Reinforce comfort measures
  - Refer to hospice and palliative care, if appropriate (Bader & Littlejohns, 2004)

Disease Expected Outcomes

- Dying is not associated with choking or smothering, but instead, it usually occurs during sleep; <1% die an uncomfortable death
- Death: average 2-5 years after diagnosis; mean 4 years extended survival
- About 15-40% live ≥ 5 years
- Another 10% live ≥ 10 years
- Poor prognosis with increasing age, severe weight loss, rapid rate of decline, no gastrostomy tube, and no ventilator support (Bader & Littlejohns, 2004)

Acquired Immune Deficiency Syndrome

AIDS (also called Auto Immunodeficiency Syndrome) is a communicable disease that develops as a result from an infection with the HIV virus (Bader & Littlejohns, 2004).

Epidemiology

- HIV infection is a global health disparity; reports estimate that in 2001, about 900,000 individuals in the U.S. were infected with the virus
- As of 2000, there has been slightly more than 806,000 reported AIDS cases in the U.S. alone
- Women are increasingly exposed to HIV transmission, although men still account for the largest population of infected
- HIV is increasing at a faster rate in Hispanic and African-American groups than in non-Hispanic whites
- Heterosexual transmission of HIV has continued to rise (Bader & Littlejohns, 2004)

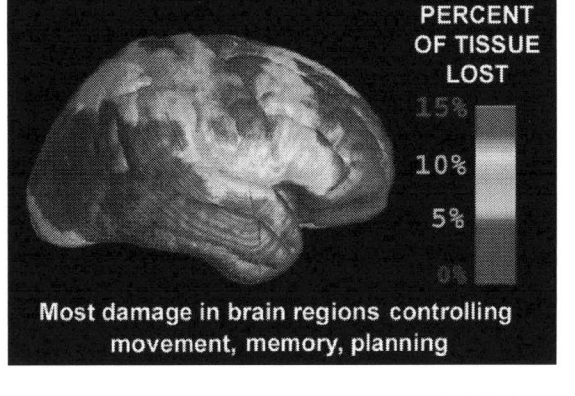

Etiology

- Known means of contracting HIV infection, thus leading to AIDS, includes sexual contact with an infected person, either vaginally or rectally, without condom protection (or by a defective condom)
- Can also be contracted through transfusions of infected blood and use of non-sterile needles
- HIV can be passed from mother to baby, although transmissions have been decreasing significantly because of *Retrovir* treatment during pregnancy
- The appearance of AIDS in HIV-infected individuals is related to CD4 helper T lymphocyte counts (Bader & Littlejohns, 2004)

Classification

- HIV is an infectious viral disease
- AIDS is a symptom complex representing complications of HIV infection, which includes opportunistic infections, certain cancers, and decreased CD4 counts (Bader & Littlejohns, 2004)

Pathophysiology

- HIV attacks all systems in the body once the individual is infected with the virus
- 15-30% of AIDS patients have direct nervous system involvement including AIDS dementia, distal symmetrical polyneuropathy (DSPN), and AIDS myelopathy

- Indirect nervous system involvement is associated with opportunistic infections that occur as a result of immune system depression caused by AIDS progression
    - Toxoplasmosis, CNS lymphoma, *C. neoformans* meningitis, progressive multifocal leukoencephalopathy, and CMV infections (Bader & Littlejohns, 2004)

Prevention

- Primary prevention is protection from contact with blood and bodily fluids of an infected individual
- Monogamous sexual relationships, use of condoms during sexual activity, and one-time use of needles can prevent the spread of HIV
- Nurses should use standard precautions with all patients for protection from infectious diseases including HIV (Bader & Littlejohns, 2004)

Assessment

- Subjective
    - In early AIDS dementia, the patient may complain of forgetting things or being unable to read or remember words and/or may complain of clumsiness, sloppy handwriting, tremor, and depressive feelings
    - In early DSPN, the patient may complain of numbness, tingling, and pain
    - In early AIDS myelopathy, the patient may complain of weakness in lower extremities
    - The early subjective signs of indirect nervous system involvement are consistent with early subjective signs of increased ICP and meningitis (Bader & Littlejohns, 2004)
- Objective
    - AIDS dementia
        - Early - memory impairment, mental slowing, depression, and gait difficulty; may forget things in middle of conversation and daily events
        - Progressive - cognitive deficits increase to the extent that the person may not be able to work or function independently
        - Severe - damage to the patient's cognition and awareness continues; by end stage, the patient has no understanding of the world, no verbalization, and no ability to care for himself/herself. At this point, the patient is under total care (Bader & Littlejohns, 2004).
    - DSPN
        - Seen in late-HIV cases
        - Dyesthesias of the feet range from mild to severe
        - Pain is worsened by touch or pressure
        - Pain impacts sleep and walking, at times
        - Symptoms move progressively and symmetrically up the feet and legs (Bader & Littlejohns, 2004)

- o AIDS myelopathy
  - Occurs in 5-10% of patients with AIDS, mostly in advanced stage of disease process
  - Gait imbalance, spastic weakness of the legs, and urinary and/or bowel incontinence are symptoms (Bader & Littlejohns, 2004)
- Diagnostics
  - o Medical history and clinical presentation
  - o Labs: for all disorders related to HIV, the CD4 cell count is needed to monitor immune deficiency
  - o CT and MRI: look for cortical atrophy
  - o For DSPN: diagnostic tests are aimed at ruling out other diseases before nerve conduction testing is completed (Bader & Littlejohns, 2004)

Treatment

- Antiretrovirals; HAART (highly active antiretroviral therapy)
- Protease inhibitors - monitor liver function
- Nutritional supplements
- Home care
- Behavior management
- TENS units (Bader & Littlejohns, 2004)

Bell's Palsy

Bell's palsy is unilateral facial paralysis that follows impairment of the facial nerve (CN VII). Bell's palsy is the most common disease of the facial nerve (Bader & Littlejohns, 2004).

Epidemiology

- Approximately 40,000 people in the U.S. per year are affected by Bell's palsy (Bader & Littlejohns, 2004).

Etiology

- No seasonal patterns or geographical or gender distinctions are seen in Bell's palsy.
- Both left and right sides of the face are affected with equal frequency.
- More prevalent in individuals with diabetes, hypertension, or influenza or other respiratory illnesses, as well as in pregnant women

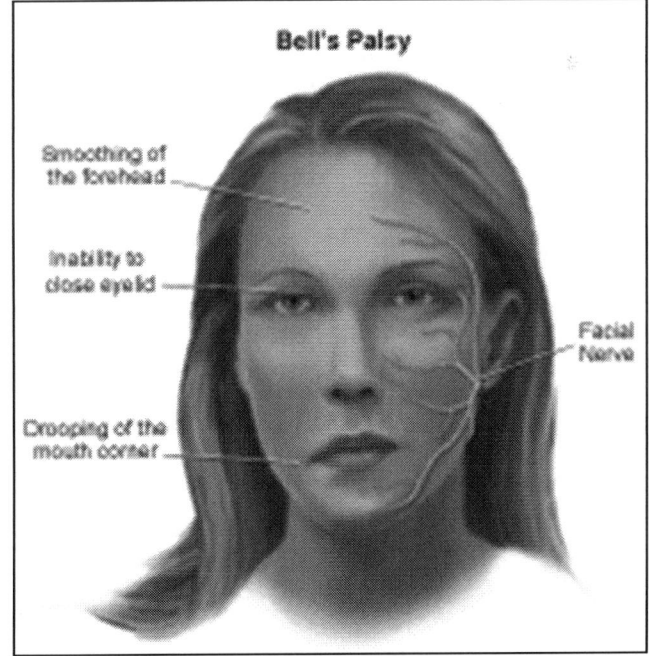

- Classification: Herpesvirus (most cases) and idiopathic (Bader & Littlejohns, 2004)

Pathophysiology

- The cause of Bell's palsy remains unknown, but is believed that most cases are a result of herpesvirus; some are idiopathic.
- Inflammation and compression of the facial nerve may be present.
- Recovery occurs quickly and without invasive interventions, thus making it difficult to study (Bader & Littlejohns, 2004).

Assessment

- Subjective
  - Patient may complain of pain behind the ear a day before the acute onset of unilateral facial weakness; maximum facial weakness occurs within 48 hours
  - Feeling of facial stiffness on the affected side
  - Decrease in taste occurs during the duration of the palsy
  - Hyperacusis - an abnormal sensitivity to sound on the affected side (Bader & Littlejohns, 2004)
- Objective
  - Paralysis is noticeable with the face at rest because of smoothing of the normal facial folds and lines on one side
  - Unilateral absence of voluntary movement of the facial muscles
  - The corneal reflex is absent
  - Salivary secretions are decreased
  - Lacrimation of the affected eye is reduced (Bader & Littlejohns, 2004)
- Diagnostics
  - Comprehensive medical history and physical: diagnosis is based primarily on the clinical presentation
  - CT or MRI: may be necessary to differentiate Bell's palsy from a tumor or vascular event
  - Electromyography: may be recommended if paralysis does not improve after 10 days to rule out a temporary conduction defect and a pathological denervation (Bader & Littlejohns, 2004)

Treatment

- Combination of steroids and antiviral agents - prednisone and acyclovir (Zovirax)
- Lubrication and patching of the affected eye are helpful
- Massage of the affected muscles may be performed
- Nursing care - routine

Outcomes

- Recovery time is a few weeks for most patients

- The return of motor function within 5 to 7 days is a good prognostic sign
- Almost 8,000 cases annually report permanent facial weakness (Bader & Littlejohns, 2004)

Encephalitis

Encephalitis is the inflammation of the brain parenchyma that is caused by a virus, bacteria, fungus, or parasite. *Viral encephalitis* is the most common and affects the cerebral hemispheres, then the brainstem. With encephalitis, there is generally altered mental status, behavior and personality changes, and speech or motor/movement or sensory deficits (Bader & Littlejohns, 2004).

Epidemiology

- Approximately 200,000 cases of acute viral encephalitis annually in the U.S.
- Mortality rate is 5-20%; 20% will have neurological deficits (Bader & Littlejohns, 2004)

Etiology

- Viruses that target CNS
    - Respiratory system is the entrance for measles, mumps, and varicella
    - Oral-intestinal route admits enteroviruses and polioviruses
    - Oral or genital mucosa is pathway for herpes simplex virus (HSV)
    - Rabies
    - Mosquito bites
    - Lyme disease
    - Transplant infection of a fetus may occur with cytomegalovirus (CMV), HIV, and rubella
    - Immunocompromised are at highest risk (Bader & Littlejohns, 2004)

Pathophysiology

The virus enters the body and colonizes; then, it penetrates the cell and transcribes and replicates the viral nucleic acid. The blood-brain barrier prevents the virus from entering the CNS. However, the virus can enter the CNS through the cerebral capillaries, peripheral nerves, or choroid plexus. In acute encephalitis, the virus attacks neurons and causes cellular lysis. In HSV and varicella zoster, the virus can become latent for long periods of time and may continue for months or years (Bader & Littlejohns, 2004).

Assessment

- Signs vary with the organism and area involved
- Headache is usually present
- Fever, nuchal rigidity, altered LOC may be present

- Other neurological changes include focal neurological deficits, aphasia, seizures, Babinski's reflex, involuntary movements, and cranial nerve deficits (Bader & Littlejohns, 2004).

Diagnostics

- Comprehensive medical history and clinical examination
- Lab studies
    - CSF studies
    - Serology
    - EEG, CT, MRI
- Surgery - tissue biopsy may be necessary in some cases

Treatment

- Treatment mirrors that for bacterial meningitis (Bader & Littlejohns, 2004)

Guillain-Barré Syndrome

Guillain-Barré is an acute, inflammatory, demyelinating polyneuropathy that causes weakness, sensory loss, and areflexia (Bader & Littlejohns, 2004).

Epidemiology

- Occurs in 1-2 out of 100,000 people per year
- Affects all ages, races, and genders equally (Bader & Littlejohns, 2004)

Etiology and Contributing Factors

- Immune mediate: humoral and cellular
- Precipitating factors: 1 to 3-week infection, usually viral, preceded 60-70% of cases
    - *Campylobacter jejuni* implicated in 24-50% of cases (Bader & Littlejohns, 2004)

Classification

- Most common is the *demyelinating* form
- Less common are *axonal* variations
- Miller Fisher syndrome
    - Rare
    - Benign
    - Triad includes: ophthalmoplegia, ataxia, and areflexia (Bader & Littlejohns, 2004)

Prevention

- There is no known prevention of this disorder other than avoidance of viral infections (Bader & Littlejohns, 2004).

Pathophysiology

- The hallmark is inflammatory lesions throughout the peripheral nervous system (PNS)
- Macrophages attack myelin (Bader & Littlejohns, 2004)

Assessment

- Subjective data
  - Rapidly progressive weakness and/or paresthesias, usually ascending
  - Onset can be over hours or days
  - Sensory loss may or may not be present; may be severe
  - Loss of deep tendon reflexes (DTRs)
  - Facial, ocular, or oropharyngeal muscles may be affected (50% will have facial diplegia)
  - Autonomic dysfunction including ileus, hypotension, hypertension, and arrhythmias can occur
  - When weakness *ascends* to the diaphragm, respiratory compromise may be present (Bader & Littlejohns, 2004)

Diagnostics

- Lumbar puncture always shows increased protein
- Electrophysiological nerve study/nerve conduction study shows slowing or conduction
  - Block in motor and sensory nerves (Bader & Littlejohns, 2004)

Treatment

- IVIG 1-2 mg/kg in divided doses over 3 to 5 days
- Therapeutic plasma exchange (TPE) performed every other day for 10 to 15 days
- Monitor for anaphylaxis, chills, and fluid overload (Bader & Littlejohns, 2004)

Nursing Interventions

- Assess vitals and neurological function frequently
- Monitor for increasing ascending weakness
- Assess respiratory function frequently
- Teach to perform ROM exercises in unaffected limbs at least four times a day
- Positional alignment
- Provide progressive mobilization

- Observe and teach the use of adaptive mobility equipment (canes, walkers, prosthesis)
- Teach safety precautions
- Acknowledge patient's fear about sudden loss of mobility and potential for permanent disability (Bader & Littlejohns, 2004)

Potential Complications

- Pain
- Contractures
- Risk for impaired skin integrity
- Risk for complications due to the hazards of immobility
- Risk for airway compromise (Bader & Littlejohns, 2004)

Disease-Specific Expected Outcomes

- All patients experience some recovery
- Some will experience residual weakness
- Most recovery occurs in the first 12 months after illness, but can continue for up to 24 months (Bader & Littlejohns, 2004)

Meningitis

Meningitis is the inflammation of the *meninges* that cover and protect the brain and spinal cord. The three primary causes of meningitis are bacterial, viral, and fungal organisms, but it can also be caused by parasites and cancer (Bader & Littlejohns, 2004). Meningitis is characterized by meningeal inflammation with *normal* cerebral function (Hayden Gephart, 2013).

Complications of Meningitis
) Communicating hydrocephalus
) Loculated CSF collections
) Subdural effusion / empyema
) Cerebral infarction
) Cerebral abscess
) Dural sinus thrombophlebitis

Bacterial Meningitis

Epidemiology

Approximately 5 out of 100,000 people are diagnosed annually in developing countries. The use of conjugate type B (Hib) vaccine and increased incidence of PCN-resistant and cephalosporin-resistant *S. pneumonia* meningitis makes antibiotic therapy challenging (Bader & Littlejohns, 2004). The leading cause of meningitis has changed from Hib to *Streptococcus pneumoniae*. The median age has increased from 15 months to 25 years in developed countries (Bader & Littlejohns, 2004).

Etiology and Contributing Factors

Causative agents include:
- Streptococcus pneumoniae, Neisseria meningitidis, Hemophilius influenza, group B streptococcus, Escherichia coli, Listeria monocytogenes, Mycobacterium tuberculosis, and Treponema pallidum (neurosyphillis)
- Pathogens that account for >80% of bacterial meningitis cases:
  - Streptococcus pneumonia = pneumococcal meningitis
  - Neisseria meningitides = meningococcal meningitis
  - Hemophilius influenza = Hib meningitis (Bader & Littlejohns, 2004)

Risk factors include:
- Immunocompromised conditions related to immune disorders, organ transplant, and antimetabolite agent therapy
- Meningeal disruption related to penetrating head trauma, surgery, CSF leak, ICP monitoring device, and external ventricular drains
- Environmental factors such as overcrowded living conditions (college dorms, day cares, travel to endemic areas) (Bader & Littlejohns, 2004)

Primary Clinical Manifestations

- Insidious onset; non-specific illness with fever, malaise, irritability, and vomiting that progresses over 2 to 4 days
- Rapidly fulminating illness that develops in <24 hours and is often associated with poor outcome (Bader & Littlejohns, 2004)

Pathophysiology

Access routes: pathogen enters the body through an open wound, mucous membranes, or infected tissue.
- Direct pathogen invasion: wounds, skull fractures, LPs, otitis media, neurosurgical procedures and devices, sinusitis, osteomyelitis
- Hematological route: septicemia-bacteremia, septic embolus, bacterial endocarditis, URI, UTI, pelvic abscess
- CSF leak: ottorhea, rhinorrhea

Infectious process: once colonization occurs, the pathogen invades tissues and the bloodstream, crosses the blood-brain barrier, and invades the subarachnoid space; then, lysis of bacteria produces exudate and meningeal inflammation, which leads to edema, vasculitis, infarctions, hydrocephalus, and increased ICP (Bader & Littlejohns, 2004).

Prevention

The Centers for Disease Control and Prevention (CDC) monitor the outbreaks of meningitis, and all cases must be reported. Chemoprophylaxis can be given to those who have come in contact with an infected person.
- Antibiotic therapy is recommended for someone who has come in contact with an infected person: Rifampin, Rocephin, Cipro

Control an epidemic of the disease
- Epidemic threshold is defined as > 15 cases per 100,000 people per week
- Chloromycetin can be administered within 4-6 weeks of an outbreak

Vaccines are recommended for those at high risk for infection or who travel to endemic countries
- Conjugate Hib
- Meningococcal vaccine
- Pneumococcal conjugate
- *Mycobacterium tuberculosis* (Bader & Littlejohns, 2004)

Assessment

Clinical manifestations are similar for bacterial, viral, and fungal meningitis. Symptoms vary with the pathogen, but are generally:
- Headache, neck, or back pain; photophobia; and malaise found in all forms
- "Classic Triad:" headache, fever, nucal rigidity
- Meningeal irritation: HA, nucal rigidity, photophobia, Kernig's sign and Brudzinski's sign
    - Kernig's sign - patient cannot extend the leg at the knee when the thigh is flexed because of stiffness in the hamstrings
    - Brudzinski's sign - clinical sign in which forced flexion of the neck elicits a reflex flexion of the hips
    - Focal neurological deficits - cranial nerve palsies, seizures, hemiparesis, and altered mental status
    - Petechial rash - present in over 50% of meningococcal cases; distinctive rash appearing as tiny red or purple "pinpricks" and progresses to purple blotches
        - Located on trunk, lower extremities, mucous membranes, and conjunctiva
        - Rapidly evolving rash is emergent and associated with poor outcomes
        - Tumbler test - drinking glass is pressed against vasculitic spots and does not fade
- Infants: presentation can be non-specific and may include irritability, whimpering, bulging fontanels, arching back with neck retractions, fever, diarrhea, refusal to eat, vacant stare, and jaundice (Bader & Littlejohns, 2004)

Diagnosis

- Comprehensive medical history
- Laboratory studies:
    - Chemistry and coagulation profiles
    - Cultures: blood, sputum, urine, nasopharyngeal, CSF, and rash aspirate
    - CSF studies: cell count, protein, glucose, cytological analysis, Gram stain
    - Serology: latex agglutination, counter-immunoelectrophoresis, ELISA, PCR
- CT of the head:
    - Prior to lumbar puncture
- Lumbar puncture:
    - Opening pressure is elevated in bacterial meningitis

- o Contraindicated include increased ICP, focal neurological deficits, coagulopathy, meningococcal septicemia, or septic shock
- Chest and sinus radiography: Sinusitis or basilar skull fracture may evident
- Electroencephalogram (EEG) will show diffuse slowing over both hemispheres (Bader & Littlejohns, 2004)

Treatment

- Antibiotic therapy - should be administered within 30 minutes of patient's arrival to the ER
- Vancomycin (Vancocin) is first line of defense because of emergence of penicillin-resistant and cephalosporin-resistant pneumococcal organisms
- Therapy is modified to combat infection once pathogen is identified
- Corticosteroid therapy (Dexamethasone)
  - o Administered before or with first antibiotic dose in children or adults with impaired LOC, impaired focal signs, or increased ICP
  - o Reduces audiological complications and neurological sequelae in children
  - o Controversial - some studies have shown that steroids reduce the ability of antibiotics to penetrate CSF
- Surgical - drainage of CNS abscesses or insertion of VP shunt to reduce hydrocephalus

Nursing Considerations

- Implement airborne precautions (respiratory isolation) for 24 hours after the start of effective antibiotic therapy
- Assess vitals and do neuro checks regularly; assess for meningeal irritation
- Monitor labs: WBC, serum electrolytes
- Administer antibiotics as prescribed - monitor peak and trough levels
- Antipyretics prn
- Institute cooling measures, if necessary (goal: afebrile at 98.6° F)
- Analgesics prn
- Administer IVF's as ordered; monitor intake and output
- Provide privacy and encourage rest
- Promote nutritional intake; encourage fluids
- Provide appropriate skin care (Bader & Littlejohns, 2004)

Potential Complications

- Waterhouse-Friderichsen syndrome (adrenal hemorrhage)
- Disseminated intravascular coagulation
- Hearing/vision loss
- Brain abscesses/subdural effusions
- Encephalitis/hydrocephalus
- Increased ICP

- Paralysis, acute respiratory distress syndrome (ARDS)
- Seizures
- Death (Bader & Littlejohns, 2004)

Viral Meningitis

Viral meningitis, also known as *aseptic meningitis*, is the most common type of meningitis. It is a clinical syndrome of meningeal inflammation in which the pathogen is not identified by diagnostic studies (Bader & Littlejohns, 2004).

Epidemiology

- More than 75,000 cases occur each year in the U.S.
- Frequently unreported because of the mild nature of the disease and the difficulty in diagnosis (Bader & Littlejohns, 2004)

Etiology and Contributing Factors

- Common causes include enteroviruses, arboviruses, and herpesviruses
- 85-90% of cases are caused by enteroviruses and occur in summer and fall (Bader & Littlejohns, 2004)

Pathophysiology

- Transmission is through fecal-oral contamination or respiratory droplets
- Patient is infectious from 3 days after contraction up to 10 days after symptoms develop; incubation period is 3 to 7 days (Bader & Littlejohns, 2004)

Prevention

- Vaccines against polio, varicella, and measles-mumps-rubella (Bader & Littlejohns, 2004)

Assessment

- Clinical symptoms are milder than bacterial, resembling influenza
- Common symptoms - headache, fever, photophobia, malaise, and nausea
- Duration is 1 to 2 weeks after onset of symptoms (Bader & Littlejohns, 2004)

Treatment

- Empiric antibiotic therapy until culture results are negative
- Acyclovir (Zovirax) may be used to treat herpesvirus type 1 and 3 or varicella-zoster
- Supportive therapy (Bader & Littlejohns, 2004)

Fungal Meningitis

- All fungal agents can produce meningitis
- Cryptococcus neoformans is the most causative agent
- Highest risk group is among immunocompromised, especially HIV patients
- Serology (antigen tests): India ink examination, latex agglutination tests, and ELISA
- Antibiotic therapy is amphotericin B and flucytosine
- Nursing interventions are the same as with other forms of meningitis (Bader & Littlejohns, 2004)

Multiple Sclerosis

Multiple sclerosis (MS) is one of the most life-altering diagnoses a person can receive. It usually strikes in the prime of life, rapidly progresses to disability, and has no cure. MS can have a strong emotional impact—not only on those diagnosed with it, but also on the family and healthcare team. Because MS is a highly variable, multifaceted disorder, nurses who care for MS patients are faced with numerous clinical challenges. Most of the challenges are unique to MS, demanding, and time-consuming. Knowledgeable nurses are positioned to assess and educate the patient and family about the disease process, assist in the alleviation of symptoms, link to appropriate resources, and help improve quality of life.

Description

Multiple sclerosis is best described as an acquired, immune-mediated, demyelinating disease of the CNS (Bader & Littlejohns, 2004). MS is characterized by multiple CNS demyelinating events separated by time and space (Hayden Gephart, 2013). With MS, there are periods of relapses and remission, or it can gradually progress to complete dysfunction (Bader & Littlejohns, 2004). The disability that results from MS is caused by focal inflammation and demyelination, which then cause conduction block. The demyelination in MS is the injury or loss, partially or completely, of the myelin sheath (Bader & Littlejohns, 2004).

MS has three different subtypes:
- Relapsing remitting (RRMS)
- Primary progressive (PPMS)
- Secondary progressive (SPMS) (Hayden Gephart, 2013)

Clinical Remission

- Resolution of inflammation, redistribution of sodium channels, and re-myelination
- Axonal degeneration is the main determinant of progressive neurological disability (Bader & Littlejohns, 2004).

Epidemiology

- U.S. prevalence is 400,000 (10,000 cases/year); global prevalence is 2.5 million
- In one year of disease, patients tend to have 1-2 clinical exacerbations with 5-10 new MRI findings
- Onset between ages 18 and 50 (70-80% of cases between 20 and 40 years old)
- 1.5 to 2 times more prevalent in females
- Occurs in more affluent, economically developed, industrialized regions that have better sanitation systems
- Women are more likely to be diagnosed earlier in life
- Men are more likely to experience a more progressive course and cumulative disability
- Caucasians are at higher risk (Bader & Littlejohns, 2004)
- High prevalence in northern European ancestry (Scandinavian) (Hayden Gephart, 2013)
- Familial incidence
  - Tenfold increase in incidence of concordance for dizygotic twins
  - 10-20% of patients have an affected family member
- Prognosis and predictors of disease course
  - *Favorable, less disabling course*: being female < 40 years old; *afferent deficits* (impaired visual acuity and sensation) as opposed to *efferent deficits* (motor and incoordination); clinically isolated event with normal MRI
- Mortality
  - Mean survival from diagnosis has changed from 6 to 14 years
  - Severe disability (7.5 on Expanded Disability Status Scale) is a predictor of major risk factor for death
  - Disability (<7.5 on Expanded Disability Status Scale) is a predictor of risk for death (Bader & Littlejohns, 2004)

Etiology

- There are no clear causes; likely a combination of causes
  - Environmental factors
    - Infectious - viral
    - Uhthoff - fever-induced conduction block
  - Candidate viruses (despite no unequivocal link)
    - Measles virus that causes encephalitis mimics MS MRI lesions
    - Canine distemper
    - Coronavirus
    - Herpes simplex virus and human herpesvirus 6
    - Chlamydia pneumonia; Epstein-Barr virus; retrovirus (human T-lymphotrophic virus 1)
  - Genetic factors
    - MS is a *polygenic* disease (runs in family); Human Leukocyte antigen (HLA)

- o Immune factors
  - Inflammatory demyelinating disease (evident on MRI showing sclerotic plaque formation)
  - Permeability of the blood-brain barrier (Bader & Littlejohns, 2004)

Symptoms

These include an episode of neurological disturbance that is likely to be inflammatory and demyelinating in nature, with clinical symptoms of >24 hours duration, with objective clinical findings, and separated by >30 days from other clinically significant events (Bader & Littlejohns, 2004).

Pathophysiology

MS is an immune-mediated, organ-specific disease of the CNS that includes inflammation, demyelination, and axonal loss (Bader & Littlejohns, 2004).

Assessment

- Subjective data
  - Clinical manifestations
    - Motor symptoms - weakness, spasticity, heaviness, stiffness of extremities
    - Somatosensory symptoms - numbness, burning, tingling, tightness, Lhermitte's sign, pain
      - Lhermitte's sign is an electrical sensation that runs down the back and into the limbs. In many patients, it is elicited by bending the head forward.
    - Brainstem symptoms - nystagmus, internuclear ophthalmoplegia (INO), dysarthria, dysphagia
    - Emotional lability
    - Visual pathway symptoms - optic neuritis, visual field defect, decreased acuity, impaired color perfection
    - Cerebellar manifestations - gait ataxia, dysmetria, intention tremor
    - Cognitive and psychiatric disturbances
    - Fatigue (present in over 90% of patients) - *worse in afternoon and evening*
    - Sleep problems
    - Bladder, bowel, and sexual disturbances
    - Paroxysmal symptoms - seizures, paroxysmal dysarthria, paroxysmal itching, trigeminal neuralgia
    - Movement disorders
    - Psychiatric and neurobehavioral syndromes
      - Cognitive dysfunction
      - Emotional disinhibition
      - Emotional lability
      - Euphoria
      - Anxiety

- Panic disorder
- Depression
- Bipolar disorder
- Motor dysfunction - muscle weakness, reflexes
  - Increased deep tendon reflexes (DTR)
  - Hyperreflexia
  - Babinski's sign
  - Hoffman's sign
  - Ankle clonus
  - Superficial abdominal reflexes frequently absent
- Spasms - extensor, flexor, usually nocturnal in nature, frequently involve limbs
- Spasticity - movement disorders, paroxysmal symptoms, seizures, sleep impairment
- Visual dysfunctions - decreased visual acuity, optic neuritis, optic pallor, afferent pupillary defect, visual field defect, scotomata

Interventions

- Relapse management
  - Pharmacological interventions include corticotropin, methylprednisolone (acute attacks), prednisone, pulse steroids, pulse cyclophosphamide, and combination
- Disease-modifying agents
  - Immunosuppresants
    - Azathioprine
    - Cyclophosphamide
    - Methotrexate
    - Mitoxantrone
  - Immunomodulating agents (used frequently during relapses)
    - Glatiramer acetate (Copaxone)
    - INF-B1a (Avonex)
    - INF-B-1a (Rebif)
    - INF B-1b (Betaseron)
    - IVIG
  - Non-pharmacological interventions
    - Rehabilitation
    - Symptom management-specific
    - Prevention measures
  - Psychosocial issues and interventions
    - Response to chronic disease
    - Emotional status
    - Support networks
    - Family and relationships
    - Pregnancy
    - Culture

- Financial
            - Vocational
            - Recreational
            - Depression and suicide
            - Potential for abuse and neglect
        - Patient advocacy
            - Patient rights
            - Ethical practices
            - Negotiating the healthcare system
            - Empowerment
            - Community resources
        - Education
            - Health promotion
            - Gender differences
            - Resources and referrals
            - Adherence
    - Objective data
        - History - demographic profile
        - Physical examination
            - Symptoms, white matter involvement, abnormal neurological examination
        - Measures of disability
            - Minimal Record of Disability (MRD) - two main functions: 1) to assist doctors and other professionals in planning and coordinating the care of people with MS; 2) to provide a standardized means of recording repeated clinical evaluations of individuals for research purposes
            - Expanded Disability Status Scale (EDSS) - a method of quantifying disability in multiple sclerosis
            - Functional Score (FS) - assesses pyramidal, cerebellar, brainstem, sensory, bowel and bladder, visual, cerebral (or mental), and other variables
            - Ambulation Index (AI) - assesses mobility by evaluating the time and degree of assistance required to walk 25 feet
            - Scripps Neurological Rating Scale
            - Multiple Sclerosis Quality of Life Inventory
            - Multiple Sclerosis Functional Composite (Bader & Littlejohns, 2004)

Diagnostics

- Based on demonstration of lesions disseminated over time and involving multiple, discrete anatomic loci in CNS white matter
- Laboratory profile
    - CSF - not indicated if history, physical, and MRI are consistent with MS; evidence of elevated IgG; presence of oligoclonal bands in CSF, but *not* in serum
    - MRI - shows 90-95% of white matter lesions in brain and 50-75% lesions in spinal cord; Gadolinium enhancement on T1 imaging

- McDonald diagnostic criteria - two attacks separated in space and time; no better explanation; specific MRI criteria; CSF findings (Bader & Littlejohns, 2004)

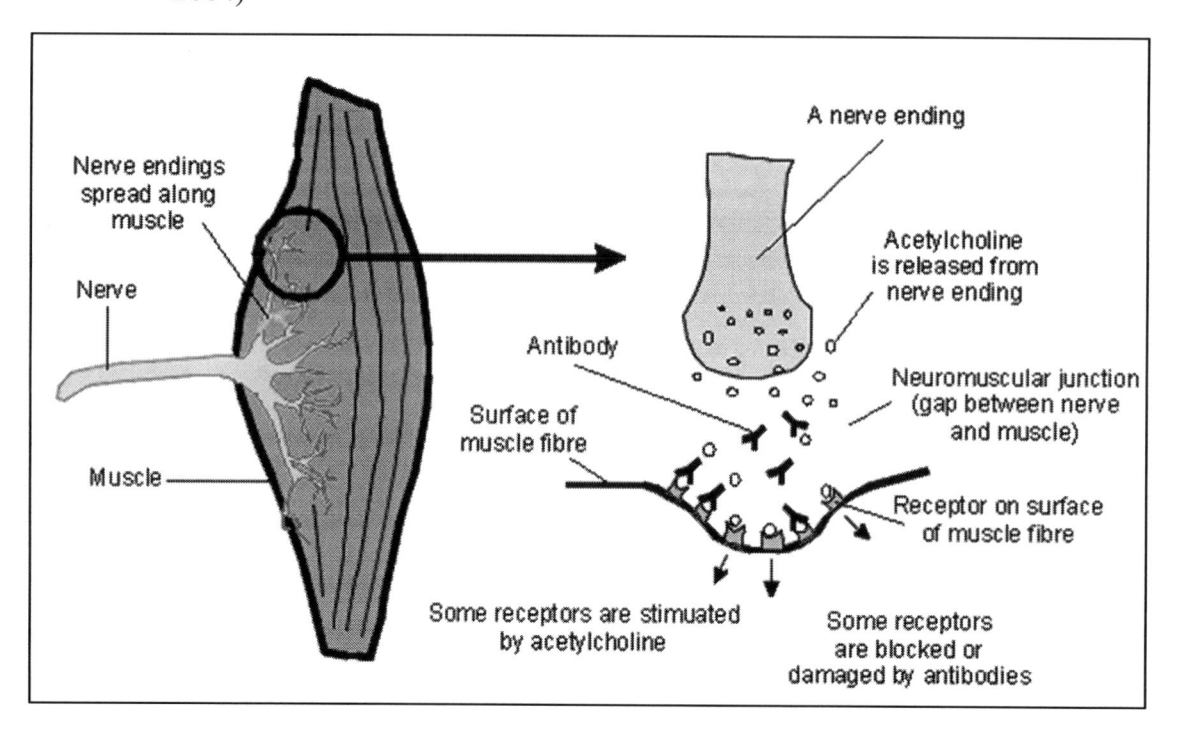

Symptom Management

In addition to starting antiviral drugs as discussed previously, patients with MS may need to be prescribed a CNS stimulant in order to combat fatigue. Drugs such as Cylert, Provigil, and Ritalin may be started. Due to the high abuse potential and side effects, patients must be routinely monitored to assess efficacy. Other drugs that treat MS symptoms include selective serotonin reuptake inhibitors (SSRIs) to combat depression and 4-Aminopyridine, a potassium channel blocker, to lower the seizure threshold. To palliate spasticity, 5 mg of Baclofen taken twice daily may be needed and can be administered orally and intrathecally. Zanaflex, Valium, Dantrium, Catapres, Neurontin, and Botulinum toxin type A also help to decrease spasticity and pain (Bader & Littlejohns, 2004).

Nursing Interventions

- Assess for UTI, other infections, and acute exacerbations
- Assess lifestyle
- Assess comorbidities and accompanying chronic diseases (DM, CHF, thyroid, etc.)
- Assess for chronic pain, sleep pattern, and nutrition and fluid intake
- Assess for level of disability and deconditioning
- Recommend energy conservation
- Prioritize/organize

- Use assistive devices
- Promote rest and sleep
- Recommend energy-enhancing resistance to fatigue: exercise, sleep, scheduled pleasurable activities, nutrition
- Encourage positive attitude
- Recommend keeping cool: cooling system, layered clothing, cold drinks
- Refer to rehabilitation and counseling (Bader & Littlejohns, 2004)

Myasthenia Gravis

Myasthenia gravis (MG) is best described as an autoimmune disorder where normal transmission of nerve impulses is interrupted at the neuromuscular junction. The disorder was first described in 1672 by Sir Thomas Willis. The disorder affects the voluntary muscle groups including ocular, oropharyngeal, facial, shoulders, girdle, and limbs. The hallmark characteristics of myasthenia gravis are fluctuating muscle weakness and fatigue that is exacerbated by exercise and improved with rest (Bader & Littlejohns, 2004).

Epidemiology

- Incidence is approximately <1.1 out of 100,000 people
- Prevalence is growing due to better understanding, improved diagnostics and treatment, and an aging population surviving other chronic diseases
- Affects all ages, but onset is usually 50 years of age and older
- 10-15% of autoimmune myasthenia occurs before age 20
- Thymus abnormalities are seen in 75% of cases
- Genetics may play a role; however, familial cases are rare
- Spontaneous remission has occurred in 10-20% of cases (Bader & Littlejohns, 2004)

Etiology and Contributing Factors

- Generally, an acquired autoimmune process
- Acetylcholine (Ach) receptors are reduced by autoantibodies, which results in impaired neuromuscular transmission and subsequent muscle weakness (Bader & Littlejohns, 2004)

Classification

- Insidious onset
- Types of MG:
  - Ocular - weakness of eye and lid muscles only
  - Bulbar - involves muscles of speech, swallowing, and breathing
  - Generalized - involves proximal muscles of upper and lower extremities, as well as ocular and/or bulbar involvement

- o Neonatal transient - transplacental passage of autoantibodies from myasthenic mother to newborn
- o Non-immune - congenital myasthenic syndromes including Lambert-Eaton myasthenic syndrome (Bader & Littlejohns, 2004)

Initial Manifestations

- Ptosis and/or diplopia in 80% of cases; weakness is limited to ocular area in 10% of patients
- Oropharyngeal weakness manifested by painless, fatigable dysphagia or dysphonia
- A small percentage have fatigable limb weakness as presenting symptom (Bader & Littlejohns, 2004)
- Characteristics of MG weakness
  - Fluctuations over time; generally increases during course of the day
  - Worsens after sustained activity/use of affected muscles
  - Exacerbations related to stress, systemic illness/infection, fever, surgery, menses, pregnancy, hypothyroidism or hyperthyroidism, heat, hypokalemia, and medications affecting neurotransmission (Bader & Littlejohns, 2004)
    - o Myasthenia Gravis Foundation of America classification system
      - Class I through Class V

Assessment

- Subjective data
  - o Muscle weakness/fatigue with sustained activity; improved with rest
  - o Diplopia and ptosis
  - o Slurred and/or nasal speech
  - o Dysphagia
  - o Shortness of breath
- Objective data
  - o Cranial nerve (CN) assessment
    - I Olfactory - olfaction (smell)
    - II Optic - vision (contains 38% of all the axons connecting to the brain)
    - III Oculomotor - eyelid and eyeball muscles
    - IV Trochlear - eyeball muscles
    - V Trigeminal - facial and mouth sensation, chewing
    - VI Abducens - eyeball movement
    - VII Facial - taste, facial muscles and salivary glands
    - VIII Auditory - hearing and balance
    - IX Glossopharyngeal - taste, swallowing
    - X Vagus - main nerve of the parasympathetic nervous system (PNS)
    - XI Accessory - moving head and shoulder
    - XII Hypoglossal - tongue muscles
  - o Screening assessment
    - Gait and legs - may have difficulty walking

- Arms, shoulder, hands - no pronator drift; grip weakness
  - Motor assessment
    - Assess position, muscle bulk, tone, strength, alternating movements, point-to-point
  - Sensory assessment - usually intact
  - Reflex assessment - usually intact
  - Mental status assessment
  - Respiratory assessment (Bader & Littlejohns, 2004)

Diagnostics

- Labs
  - Anti-AChR antibody test
  - Thyroid function screening to rule out hypothyroidism and hyperthyroidism
- Electromyography
- Tensilon test - use anticholinesterase inhibitor given intravenously and assess for improved strength of muscles after 45-60 seconds
- CT scan of mediastinum to assess thymus (Bader & Littlejohns, 2004)

Treatment

- Treated with anticholinesterase inhibitor
- Pyridostigmine bromide (Mestinon) most commonly prescribed
- Corticosteroids - may take 6-8 weeks to attain maximum benefits
- Immunosuppressive agents - Imuran; maximum benefit in 3 to 12 months
- Cyclosporine - Neoral; inhibits T cell response; 1-2 months improvement after initiation; maximum benefit in 6 months
- IVIG - mechanism not well understood
- CellCept - for organ transplant immunosuppression
- Surgery - thymectomy; maximum response in 2 to 5 years (Bader & Littlejohns, 2004)

Nursing Interventions

- Assess effect of drug interventions
- Advise patient of drug side effects
  - Mestinon - GI upset, bronchial secretions, miosis, muscle cramps, weakness, fasiculations
  - Corticosteroids - weight gain, emotional lability, GI upset or ulcer, insomnia, fluid retention
- Note time of day patient is weakest
- Assist patient in achieving optimal activities of daily living (ADL) goals
- Educate about energy conservation (Bader & Littlejohns, 2004)

Chapter 5: Seizure Disorders

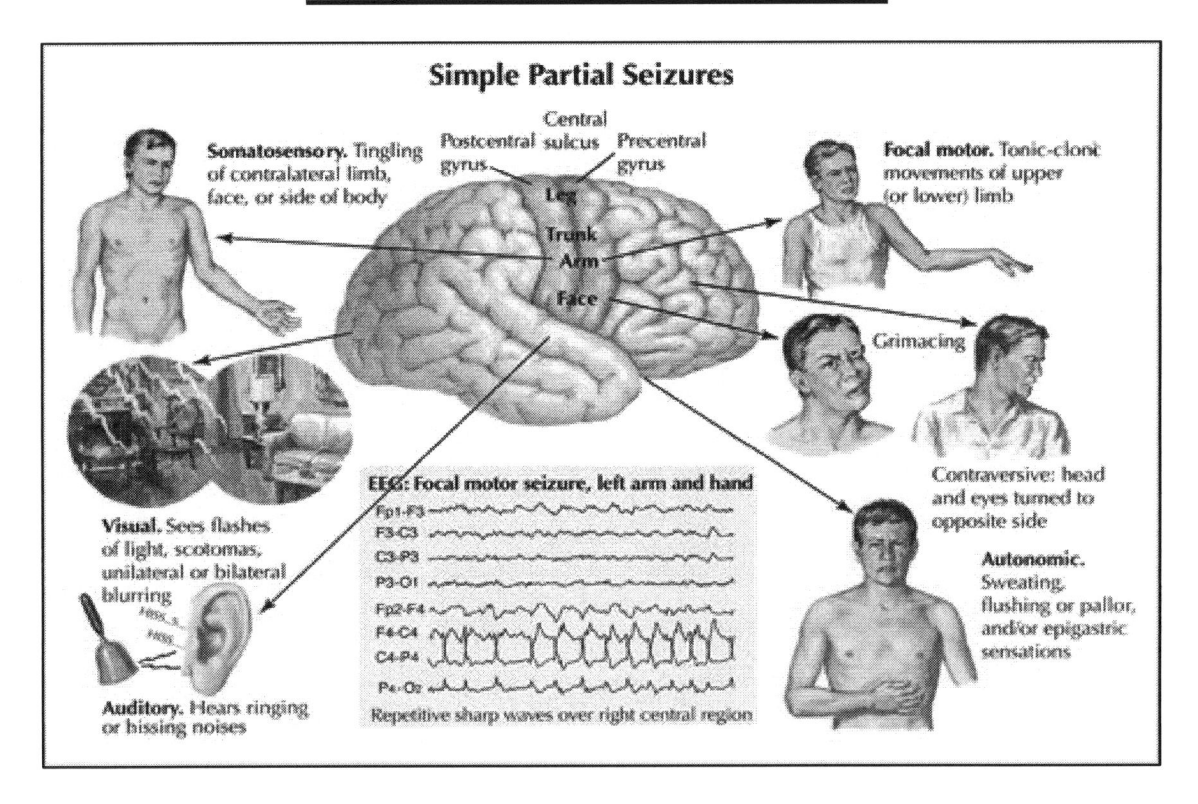

A seizure can be described as a clinical manifestation of the central nervous system (CNS) that is characterized by abnormal electrical firing within the brain. The characteristics of seizures depend on the location of the epileptiform transients. *Epilepsy* is the condition in which there is recurrence of unprovoked seizures secondary to biochemical, anatomical, and physiological changes and variables (Bader & Littlejohns, 2004). Patients with epilepsy have recurrent seizures with correlating clinical symptoms and EEG findings (Hayden Gephart, 2013).

Etiology

Seizures can be related to numerous causative factors and disorders:
- Idiopathic or a result of unknown cause
- Cryptogenic or related to a presumed cause that is ill-defined
- Symptomatic as a result of a known cerebral abnormality or insult
  - Cerebral trauma - seizures more prominent if there is an LOC > 30 minutes
  - Lesions that compete for intracerebellar space (tumors, AV malformations, subdural hematomas)
- Neurofibromatosis may precipitate seizures
- Cerebral infections (meningitis, encephalitis, abscess)
  - Aseptic meningitis patients are at less risk for seizures
- Febrile convulsions are associated with the development of epilepsy
- Genetic factors such as chromosomal abnormalities

- Thrombolytic or hemorrhagic stroke
- Hypoxic acidosis
- Alzheimer's disease
- Familial history
- Metabolic disorders (Bader & Litttlejohns, 2004)

Epidemiology

Approximately 10% of the population will experience a single, unprovoked seizure in their lifetime (Hayden Gephart, 2013). Generalized seizures are mainly age-dependent and occur within the first five years of life. The occurrence of partial seizures increases with age (Bader & Littlejohns, 2004). There are several comorbidities related to epilepsy:

- Mental retardation and developmental delay (28-38% of children with epilepsy)
- Depression and mood disorders occur in 20% of patients with epilepsy diagnosis
- Sudden, unexplained death occurs more in patients with epilepsy diagnosis than in those without
- Memory impairment
- Headaches (Bader & Littlejohns, 2004)

Pathophysiology

Seizure activity occurs when brain cells become abnormally linked together. Generally, seizures arise from an imbalance between cerebral excitation and inhibition. Activity may be related to a loss of cells that inhibit excitatory cells or when there are an overabundant number of excitatory cells.
- Excitation - Glutamate is the most important excitatory neurotransmitter involved with epilepsy
- Inhibition - GABA drives activity of Cl^-, Ca^{++}, and K^+ channels (Bader & Littlejohns, 2004)

Classifications of Seizures

The International Classification of Epileptic Seizures classifies each individual seizure based on electroencephalography (EEG) and clinical data. This classification system provides a common clinical language in which to describe and document seizures (Bader & Littlejohns, 2004).

- Partial - onset of synchronous cortical discharges involving the focal brain region
- Simple Partial - sudden onset of synchronous cortical discharges resulting in associated symptoms specific to the brain region affected, but without alteration in LOC. An "aura" is a simple partial.
  o Facial twitching or hand jerking
  o Somatosensory events (unusual taste in mouth)
  o Autonomic events like vomiting, diaphoresis, and epigastric sensation
  o "Psychic" events such as illusions, hallucinations, and déjà vu may occur

Classification of Seizures

Partial (or Focal) Seizures

- **Simple Partial**
  - Awareness <u>not</u> impaired
- **Complex Partial**
  - Awareness impaired/lost
- **Partial Seizures secondarily generalizing**

Generalized Seizures

- **Absence**
  - Typical
  - Atypical
- **Myoclonic**
- **Clonic**
- **Tonic**
- **Tonic-Clonic**
- **Atonic**

- Complex Partial - onset of synchronous cortical discharges resulting in associated symptoms specific to the brain region affected, but with alteration in LOC
  - May or may not be preceded by simple partial seizures; most common type
  - Automatisms such as lip smacking, blinking, and picking at clothing occur
  - Motor phenomena such as wandering, running, and arm jerking are often associated with frontal lobe seizures
- Generalized - sudden onset of synchronous cortical discharges involving both cerebral hemispheres
- Status Epilepticus - unremitting or repeated seizure activity without interictal return to baseline
  - Seizure > 30 minutes
  - Diagnosis on EEG
  - Neuron death occurs 30-60 minutes after continuous seizure activity
  - 22% mortality rate; in coma patients, 70-80%
  - May trigger trauma, rhabdomylosis, airway compromise, cardiac failure, or pulmonary edema
  - Management: ABCs, oxygen, finger stick glucose; administer benzos first; IV Fosphenytoin; Phenytoin for oral route; Valproic acid; Versed and Propofol with high dose phenobarbital to reduce recurrence
- Pseudoseizures - Pseudoseizures are alterations in behavior that resemble seizures, but are without any organic cause. Most patients include returning war veterans, mothers in child-custody battles, and over-extended professionals. These are also called psychogenic non-epileptic seizures (PNES). The display of uncontrollable movements, far-off stares, and convulsions are not the result of abnormal electrical discharges in the brain that characterize epilepsy, but instead appear to be stress-related behaviors that mimic seizures and that are misdiagnosed as the neurological disorder (Bader & Littlejohns, 2004).

Chapter 6: Developmental and Degenerative Disorders

Developmental and degenerative disorders are oftentimes accompanied by other sequelae and are also oftentimes misunderstood. The hallmark of degenerative disorders of the CNS is the progressive loss of previously acquired abilities. In pediatric patients, a deceleration in the rate of development is often the first presentation: the child falls progressively behind other children and subsequently loses previously acquired milestones. When the declining developmental quotient is not due to an extrinsic agent or event or to secondary involvement of the CNS by a generalized systemic disease, neurodegenerative disease is considered. The same is true for the elderly. When aging adults begin to lose function of lifelong abilities, they are reaching the end of the lifecycle and will require as much care as infants and children. Nurses can aid in assessing and identifying such disorders that affect all age groups across the continuum of care.

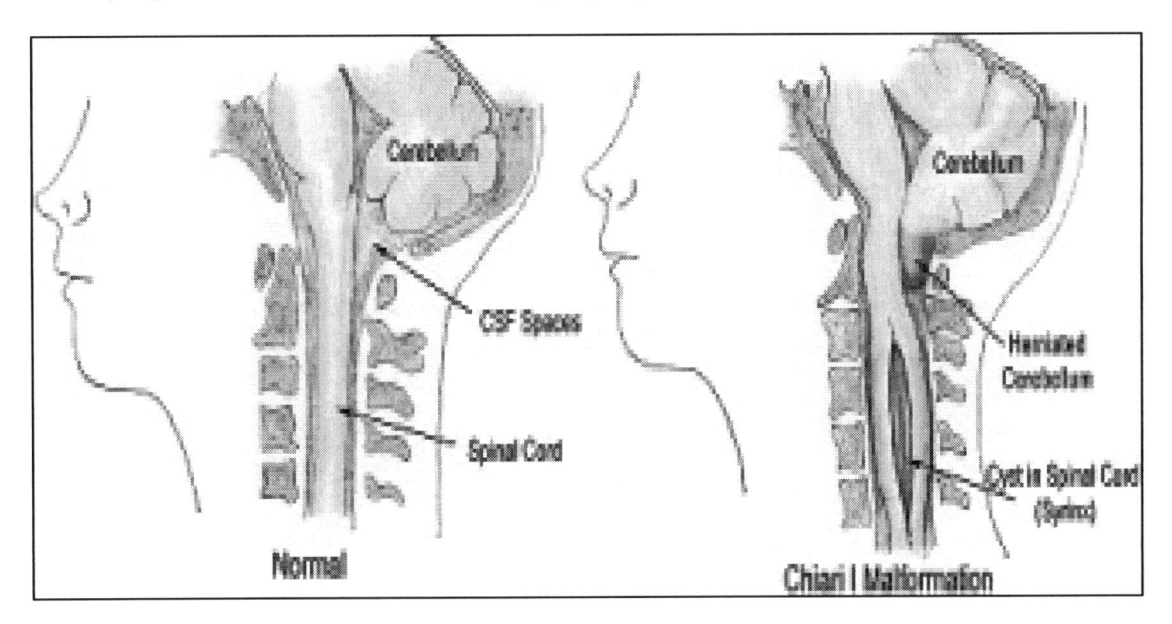

Arnold-Chiari Malformation

A Chiari malformation (CM) is a complex neuroskeletal deformity that is characterized by caudal descent of the cerebellar tonsil past the level of the foramen magnum. A Chiari malformation is often the leading cause of *syringomyelia* (a disorder in which a cyst forms within the spinal cord). This expands and elongates over time, destroying a portion of the spinal cord from its center and expanding outward (Bader & Littlejohns, 2004).

Epidemiology

- True incidence of malformation in general public is unknown
- The ratio is four females to one male
- Generally diagnosed in the third or fourth decade of life, but earlier diagnosis in infants, children, and adults is becoming more prevalent

- Considered a congenital disorder; however, post-traumatic cases have been seen (Bader & Littlejohns, 2004)

Classifications

- <u>Type I</u> - This anatomic abnormality causes the lower part of the cerebellum to protrude from its normal location in the back of the head into the cervical or neck portion of the spinal canal; commonly diagnosed in adulthood.
- <u>Type II</u> - Also called a *classic CM*, this involves the extension of both cerebellar and brainstem tissue into the foramen magnum. Also, the cerebellar vermis (the nerve tissue that connects the two halves of the cerebellum) may be only partially complete or absent. A type II is usually accompanied by a myelomeningocele—a form of spina bifida that occurs when the spinal canal and backbone do not close before birth, causing the spinal cord and its protective membrane to protrude through a sac-like opening in the back ("Chiari Malformation Fact," 2013).
- <u>Type III</u> - Diagnosed at birth and considered rare and severe, this is associated with high-level cervical meningocele, often containing neural tissue. A type III CM is associated with a very poor prognosis (Bader & Littlejohns, 2004; National Institute of Neurological Disorders and Stroke, 2013).

Pathophysiology

CMs may develop when the bony space is smaller than normal, causing the cerebellum and brainstem to be pushed downward into the foramen magnum and into the upper spinal canal. The resulting pressure on the cerebellum and brainstem may affect functions controlled by these areas and block the flow of cerebrospinal fluid (CSF) to and from the brain (National Institute of Neurological Disorders and Stroke, 2013).

Assessment

- Subjective
    - May present with a myriad of vague and transient symptoms
    - Headache - may worsen with Valsalva's maneuver, bending, or flexion of the neck
    - Dizziness
    - Weakness, numbness, and tingling of an extremity - generally unilateral
    - Fatigue
    - Pain in neck, back, and upper/lower extremities
    - Dysphagia
    - Shortness of breath

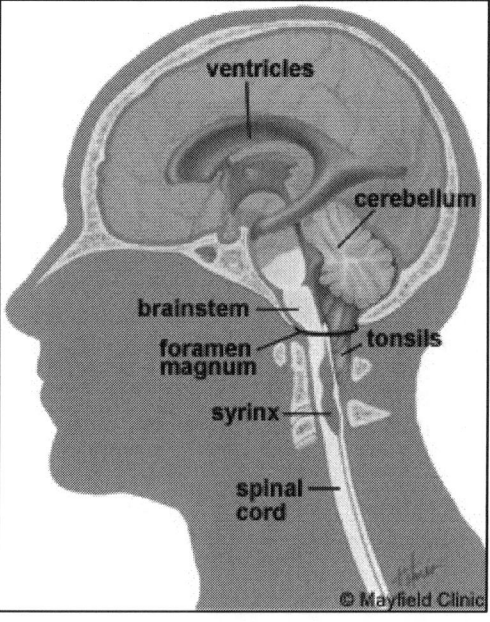

- o Neuro-ophthalmological symptoms: blurred vision, diplopia, scotomata, vision loss
- o Neuro-otic: tinnitus, hearing loss, whooshing sounds, or clicking sounds; are either unilateral or bilateral
- Objective
  - o Many have a normal neurological exam
  - o Cranial nerve assessment may be normal (Bader & Littlejohns, 2004; National Institute of Neurological Disorders and Stroke, 2013)

Diagnostics

- MRI of the brain without contrast is the first test of choice (Bader & Littlejohns, 2004).

Treatment & Interventions

- Surgical: for patient with evidence of CM on MRI and who has correlating symptoms, an elective decompression surgery may be performed - posterior fosa craniotomy, cervical laminectomy, and duraplasty
  - o Must be monitored in the ICU or step-down areas for 24 hours post-op
  - o PCA for pain control, antispasmodics, non-steroidal anti-inflammatory drugs, and antiemetics to control post-op nausea. Neurological exams must be conducted hourly for the first 24 hours. The majority of patients do very well after surgery (Bader & Littlejohns, 2004).

Outcomes

- Post-op patients are generally hospitalized for 3 to 4 days
- A follow-up MRI is obtained within 2 to 3 months
- Good prognosis (Bader & Littlejohns, 2004)

Potential Complications

- The most common post-operative complication is a pseudomeningocele (abnormal collection of CSF)
- In some instances, a post-op CSF leak occurs, which may require a lumbar drain
- Other complications include meningitis, intraoperative neurological damage, infection, and damage to major vessels (Bader & Littlejohns, 2004).

Cerebral Palsy

Cerebral palsy (CP) is a group of disorders that affect a patient's ability to move and maintain balance and posture. CP is the most common motor disability in childhood. CP is caused by abnormal brain development or damage to the developing brain that affects a person's ability to control his/her muscles (Centers for Disease Control and Prevention, 2013).

Types of Cerebral Palsy

Spastic CP

- The most common type of CP, spastic CP affects about 80% of CP patients.
  - People with spastic CP have increased muscle tone. This means their muscles are stiff and, as a result, their movements can be awkward.
  - Spastic CP is usually described by which parts of the body are affected:
    - <u>Spastic diplegia/diparesis</u> - In this type of CP, muscle stiffness is mainly in the legs, with the arms less affected or not affected at all. People with spastic diplegia might have difficulty walking because tight hip and leg muscles cause their legs to pull together, turn inward, and cross at the knees (also known as scissoring).
    - <u>Spastic hemiplegia/hemiparesis</u> - This type of CP affects only one side of a person's body; usually, the arm is more affected than the leg.
    - <u>Spastic quadriplegia/quadriparesis</u> - Spastic quadriplegia is the most severe form of spastic CP and affects all four limbs, the trunk, and the face. People with spastic quadriparesis usually cannot walk and often have other developmental disabilities such as intellectual disability; seizures; and problems with vision, hearing, or speech (Centers for Disease Control and Prevention, 2013).

Dyskinetic Cerebral Palsy (includes athetoid, choreoathetoid, and dystonic cerebral palsies)

- People with dyskinetic CP have problems controlling the movement of their hands, arms, feet, and legs, making it difficult to sit and walk. The movements are uncontrollable and can be slow and writhing or rapid and jerky. Sometimes, the face and tongue are affected, and the person has a hard time sucking, swallowing, and talking. A person with dyskinetic CP has muscle tone that can change (varying from too tight to too loose) not only from day to day, but also during a single day (Centers for Disease Control and Prevention, 2013).

Ataxic Cerebral Palsy

- People with ataxic CP have problems with balance and coordination. They might be unsteady when they walk. They might have a hard time with quick movements or movements needing a lot of control such as writing. They might have a hard time controlling their hands or arms when they reach for something.

Mixed Cerebral Palsy

- Some people have symptoms of more than one type of CP. The most common type of mixed CP is spastic-dyskinetic CP ("Facts About Cerebral," 2013).

Causes and Risk Factors

CP is caused by abnormal development of the brain or damage to the developing brain that affects a child's ability to control his/her muscles. There are several possible causes of the abnormal development or damage. People used to think that CP was caused mainly by lack of oxygen during birth. The current prevailing opinion is that brain damage that leads to CP can occur before birth, during birth, within a month after birth, or during the first years of a child's life while the brain is still developing. CP related to brain damage that occurred before or during birth is called congenital CP. The majority of CP (85-90%) is congenital. In many cases, the specific cause is not known. A small percentage of CP is caused by brain damage that occurs more than 28 days after birth. This is called *acquired CP* and is usually associated with an infection (such as meningitis) or head injury (Centers for Disease Control and Prevention, 2013).

Screening and Diagnosis

Diagnosing CP at an early age is important to the well-being of children and their families. Diagnosing CP involves several steps:
- Developmental Monitoring - also called surveillance; means tracking a child's growth and development over time. If any concerns about the child's development are raised during monitoring, a developmental screening test should be given as soon as possible.
- Developmental Screening - during developmental screening, a short test is given to see if the child has specific developmental delays such as motor or movement delays. If the results of the screening test are significant, the doctor will make referrals for developmental and medical evaluations.
- Developmental and Medical Evaluations - the goal of a developmental evaluation is to diagnose the specific type of disorder that affects a child (Centers for Disease Control and Prevention, 2013).

Treatments and Intervention Services

There is no known cure for CP, but treatment can improve the lives of diagnosed patients. It is important for patients to begin a treatment program as early as possible. After a CP diagnosis is made, a multidisciplinary team works with the child and family to develop a plan to help the child reach his/her full potential. Common treatments include medicines; surgery; braces; and physical, occupational, and speech therapy. No single treatment is best for all children with CP (Centers for Disease Control and Prevention, 2013).

Hydrocephalus

Hydrocephalus is best described as a progressive dilatation of the ventricular system due to impaired absorption of CSF. Hydrocephalus is a *clinical syndrome*, not a true entity (Bader & Littlejohns, 2004).

Epidemiology

- Congenital hydrocephalus occurs in 4-5 out of 1,000 live births
- Normal pressure hydrocephalus (NPH) is the most frequent in patients >60 years of age and is likely to remain underdiagnosed (Bader & Littlejohns, 2004)

Etiology

- Congenital-neonatal developmental anomaly; nural tube defects; genetic disorders; intrauterine infections; intracranial structural abnormalities; idiopathic
- Acquired hydrocephalus - develops sometimes after birth
    - Aqueduct of Sylvius stenosis
    - Intracranial hemorrhages
    - Infection
    - Obstructive lesion (tumor, cyst)
    - Chiari's malformation
    - Trauma/swelling
    - Superior sagittal sinus thrombosis
    - Loss of brain mass in age-related and disease-related entities, causing dilatation (Bader & Littlejohns, 2004)

Prevention

- Prenatal care and regular prenatal visits
- Post-traumatic observation for signs/symptoms of developing hydrocephalus
- Not all hydrocephalus disease processes are preventable

Classification

- Communicating - defect in the absorption of CSF at the arachnoid villi/sagittal sinus due to subarachnoid hemorrhage, infection, or gradual dysfunction due to age
    - NPH is a specific from of communicating hydrocephalus
    - Seen in older patient populations
- Obstructive - also called non-communicating hydrocephalus
    - Blockage that occurs at or above the fourth ventricle
    - Most common in aqueduct of Sylvius
    - Related to intraventricular hemorrhages, intraventricular tumors, cysts, infection, and trauma/cerebral edema (Bader & Littlejohns, 2004)

Assessment

- Subjective
    - Infants are generally difficult to console, extremely lethargic, anorexic
    - Toddler/young children with macrocephaly are often irritable, lethargic, have poor intake, have a failure to thrive, seizures

- "Classical Triad:" confusion/dementia, decreased interpersonal interaction, memory loss, loss of coordination or balance (Bader & Littlejohns, 2004)
- Objective
  - With infants, fontanel assessment when sitting upright and quiet
  - Adults: classic triad, decreased LOC, motor weakness, and signs of increased ICP (Bader & Littlejohns, 2004)

Diagnostics

- CT scan
  - Without contrast - normally adequate to assess ventricles and intracranial structures
  - With contrast - to rule out tumor, infection, and other lesions
- MRI
  - Shows greater anatomical detail
- Sonography/Ultrasound - useful primarily for neonates
- Lumbar puncture - demonstrates opening CSF pressure; generally, a transient improvement after LP and removal of CSF; avoid in patients with markedly increased ICP (risk for brainstem herniation)
- Radioisotope cisternography
- Continuous CSF drainage - placement of lumbar drain (remove approximately 5 to 10 ml/hr)
- Cine phase contrast MRI - gives good detail of third ventricle
- Prenatal ultrasound can determine diagnosis before birth (Bader & Littlejohns, 2004)

Operative Procedures

- Ventricular catheter
- Shunt valve
- Rarely used: ventriculoatrial shunt and lumboperitoneal shunts
- Endoscopic third ventriculostomy - hole is drilled into third ventricle to allow CSF to flow in the basal cisterns
  - Avoided in children under 2 years of age
  - Five-year patency rates (Bader & Littlejohns, 2004)

Nursing Considerations

- ICU admission may be necessary if neurological impairment requires intensive nursing interventions; post-op care
- Perform frequent neurological examinations for change in LOC
- Monitor for signs and symptoms of increased ICP
- FOC measurements in babies
- Educate about risk for infection (high risk for Staphylococcus epidermis and Staphylococcus aureus)
- Provide analgesics as needed

- Educate about signs and symptoms of catheter dislodgement
- Educate family that patient will have to avoid high-velocity contact sports/activities (football or karate)
- Educate on the risk of seizures
- Offer support to family over concerns (independence, learning disabilities, and special educational services) (Bader & Littlejohns, 2004)

Spina Bifida: Myelomeningocele

Spina bifida is due to a neural tube defect. There is a failure of complete closure of the neural tube. The defect can be open (aperta) or closed (occulta).

- Epidemiology - In the U.S., spina bifida is prevalent in 1 out of 1,000 births
  o Occurs during first month of pregnancy
  o Generally, no family history
  o Female prevalence
  o Highest occurrence in Welsh, Irish, and Scottish descent
- Etiology
  o Multifactorial: genetic and environmental
  o High risk if previous pregnancy with spina bifida
  o Inadequate folic acid intake
- Prevention
  o Eliminate risk factors
  o Ingest adequate folic acid - suggested to take one month prior to pregnancy
- Assess lesion site
- Serum alphafetoprotein at 16 to 18 weeks - elevated level detects an open neural tube with 75% sensitivity

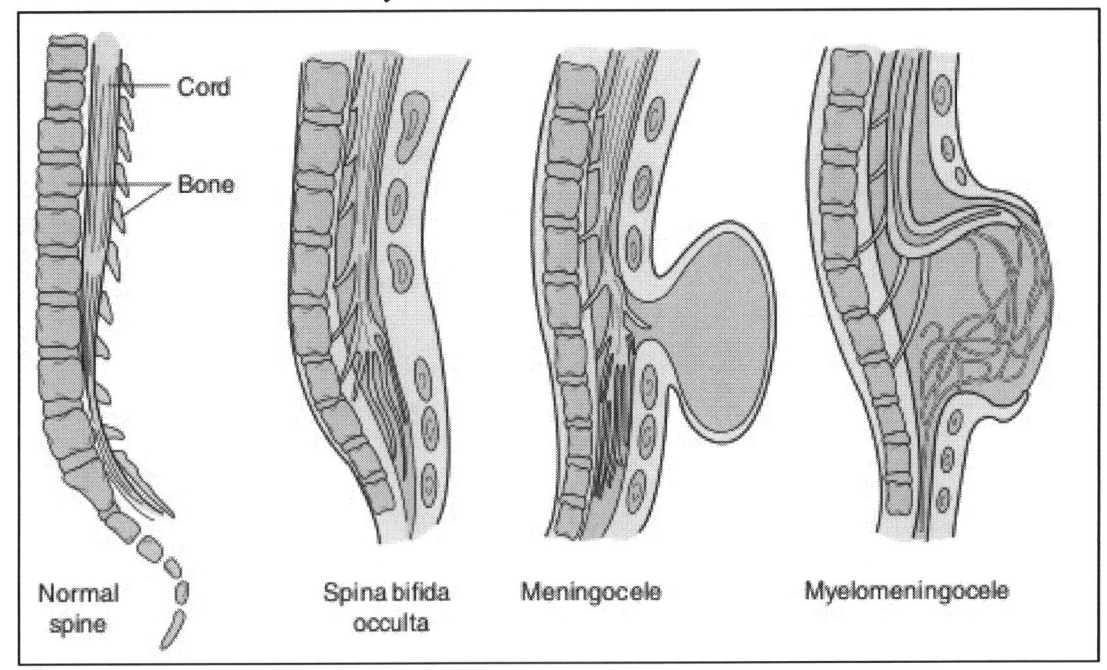

- Amniocentesis

- Prenatal ultrasound
- Maternal MRI (Bader & Littlejohns, 2004)
- Nursing care
  - Monitor site for infection in neonate
  - Monitor bowel and bladder function - assess urinary output
  - Prevent infection
  - Monitor skin integrity
  - Frequent neurological exams post-birth
  - Implement measures in order to assist patient in reaching maximum potential without losing neurological function
  - Connect family to appropriate resources (Bader & Littlejohns, 2004)

Down's Syndrome

Down's syndrome, also called Trisomy 21, is a condition in which extra genetic material causes delays in the way a child develops, both mentally and physically. It affects about 1/800 babies born in the U.S. Down's syndrome is the most common cause of mental retardation. Classical signs/symptoms of Down's syndrome include epicanthal folds, protruding tongue, transverse palmar crease, sandal sign, and hypotonia. Complications from Down's syndrome include congenital heart disease, atlanto-axial instability, GI anomalies, leukemia, immune deficiency, sleep apnea, and Alzheimer's (Hayden Gephart, 2013).

Attention Deficit Hyperactivity Disorder

Attention deficit hyperactivity disorder (ADHD) is a problem of being unable to focus, being overactive, being unable to control behavior, or a combination of these. For these problems to be diagnosed as ADHD, they must be out of the normal range for a person's age and development (David, 2013).

Diagnostic Characteristics

Symptoms present by age 7 and must cause impairment in at least two settings (home/school) with evidence of significant impairment in social/occupational functioning
- At least six of the following symptoms of inattention must have persisted for at least six months:
  - Poor attention to detail
  - Difficulty sustaining attention
  - Poor listening
  - Failure to finish projects
  - Difficulty organizing tasks
  - Avoiding sustained mental attention tasks
  - Losing important objects
  - Forgetful in daily activities

- At least six of the following symptoms of hyperactivity-impulsivity must have persisted for at least six months to a degree that is maladaptive and inconsistent with developmental level:
    - Fidgeting
    - Leaving seat frequently
    - Restlessness
    - Difficulty with quiet activities
    - Always "on-the-go"
    - Excessive talking
    - Blurting out answers
    - Difficulty taking turns
    - Interrupting
- Differential
    - Medical conditions (sleep apnea, metabolic, epilepsy)
    - Family dynamics
    - Understimulating environment
    - Oppositional or anti-social behavior
    - Result of a substance (intoxication or withdrawal)
    - Miscellaneous psychiatric disorder
- Workup
    - Psychological testing (best to involve the child, parents, teachers)
    - Consider sleep studies
- Treatment
    - Psychotherapy/family therapy
    - Stimulants (methylphenidate, mixed amphetamine salts)
    - Guanfacine, Clonidine
    - Bupropion
    - Modafinil (Hayden Gephart, 2013)
- Nursing Considerations
    - Nurses working with children and families can serve as educators to families, advocates for children, and supporters to members of the school system. When a strong, trusting relationship is built between families and nurses, parents tend to seek advice from them and rely on them to provide guidance as they manage the child's symptoms while trying to maintain a healthy, happy family life.
    - Nurses have an important role to increase community awareness about adult ADHD. Those who work in emergency rooms and in employee healthcare may be able to intervene on behalf of ADHD adults by providing education and insight to others in the environment.

Dementia

Dementia is a highly evident health disparity in the U.S. A person diagnosed with dementia can be taxing on primary caregivers and the healthcare system. Due to the growing number of aging baby boomers, dementia is highly prevalent among the general population. Nurses must be aware of the strain that can result from caring for dementia patients. Most caregivers continue to work and care for their own families while attempting to care for those diagnosed with dementia.

- Definition: Dementia is defined as intellectual deterioration severe enough to interfere with occupations and/or social performance.
- Essential Features: Impairment in short-term and long-term memory associated with impairment in abstract thinking, judgment, and other higher cortical features (Bader & Littlejohns, 2004)

Epidemiology

- Alzheimer's disease (AD) is the most common type of dementia, representing 75% of cases; there are 4.5 million people with AD.
- Prevalence doubles every 5 years between the ages of 65 and 85
- Lifetime risk: 25.5% for men; 31.9% for women
- Women are more likely to be affected by AD
- Men are more likely to be affected by vascular dementia
- Average survival from time of symptom appearance is 10.3 years (age strongly influences survival time) (Bader & Littlejohns, 2004)

Etiology

- Risk factors
  - Age and gender
  - Formal education
  - Family history
  - Genetics: Amyloid precursor protein, presenilin-1 and presenilin-2, and apolipoprotein E
  - Maternal age/Down's syndrome
  - Vascular disease (HDL ≤ 40)
- Possible protective factors
  - Estrogen
  - NSAIDs
  - Antioxidants (E and C)
  - Statins
- Reduction in choline acetyltransferase and other neurotransmitters

Prevention

- There are multiple proposed prevention measures that mostly help in slowing the onset of symptoms, not the disease process
- Estrogen exposure
- NSAIDs
- Antioxidant exposure
- Ginkgo
- Statins

- Exercise
- Social and leisure activities (Bader & Littlejohns, 2004)

Pathophysiology (AD)

- Brain atrophy: symmetric atrophy, hippocampus shrinkage, shrunken gyri, widened sulci, enlarged ventricles, thick leptomeninges
- Degenerative changes: neuritic plaques, neurofibrillary tangles, neuronal loss, amyloid protein deposits (Bader & Littlejohns, 2004)

Classification

- AD is the most common type
- Vascular dementia is a clinical syndrome of acquired intellectual impairment resulting from brain injury due to cerebrovascular disease; second most common
- Parkinson's dementia
- Lewy body's dementia
- Degenerative disorder-related dementia (Huntington's, MS, and progressive supranuclear palsy) (Bader & Littlejohns, 2004)

Clinical Sequelae

- Early stage
  - Mini-mental status examination (MMSE) scores of 26 to 30
  - Mild memory loss; confusion
  - Inability to learn new information
  - Language problems
  - Affect changes
- Middle stage
  - MMSE scores of 16 to 26
  - Profound memory loss
  - Loss of judgment
  - Lack of recognition
  - Loss of learned socially acceptable behavior
  - Personality changes
  - Loss of skilled, purposeful movement
- Late stage
  - MMSE scores of 0 to 16
  - Severe cognitive impairment
  - Physical impairments
  - Loss of self-care ability (Bader & Littlejohns, 2004)

Assessment

- Subjective
  - Early-stage patients are often aware of deficits, but not the extent of those deficits
  - Middle-stage patients often unaware of deficits and personal limitations (high safety risk)
  - Late-stage patients unable to communicate effectively with those around them
- Objective
  - Short-term and long-term memory loss
  - Confusion
  - Inability to handle ADLs such as cooking, banking, bathing
  - Personality changes
- Diagnostic
  - CT scan shows general atrophy, enlarged ventricles
    - Single-photon CT scan done in early/mild stages for hippocampus assessment
  - MRI scan: performed if there is a high suspicion of vascular involvement
  - Labs to rule out other dementia causes: CBC, Thyroid profile, Sedimentation rate, VDRL, Vitamin B12
  - Positron emission tomography (PET) scan: done mostly for research purposes; can also evaluate brain metabolism of glucose
- Cognitive evaluation tools
  - Mini-Mental Status Exam - "gold standard" used to evaluate dementia; primary outcome measure in most clinical trials to treat dementias
  - Clock-drawing evaluation - clients are asked to draw a clock face, mark the hours, and draw the hands to indicate a particular time; the CDT assesses frontal and temporo-parietal functioning
  - Blessed Dementia Rating Scale
  - Clinician's Interview-Based Impression of Change
  - Beck Depression Inventory - 21-item, self-report rating inventory that measures characteristic attitudes and symptoms of depression (Bader & Littlejohns, 2004)

Operative Procedures

- Performed only if there is an operative contributor to the dementia (brain tumor)
- Intracranial shunt procedure is very controversial, but may be helpful (Bader & Littlejohns, 2004)

Interventions

- Cholinesterase inhibitors
  - Donepezil hydrochloride (Aricept), rivastigmine (Exelon), and galantamine (Reminyl) may be administered
    - Mostly effective if started in early/middle stages

- Slows cognitive decline and manages behavior
- 5-mg Aricept tablet per day for 4 to 6 weeks, then increase to a 10-mg tablet daily
    - Side effects include insomnia (if given at night), anxiety, and nausea
- Exelon is 1.5 mg twice daily to begin, then titrate up to 6 mg twice daily
    - Must be slowly titrated over weeks to months
    - Must be taken with food to reduce significant GI upset
    - Available in transdermal patch for administration
- Reminyl is 4 mg twice a day with slow titration up to 12 mg twice per day
    - Given with food to reduce the side effects of nausea, vomiting, and diarrhea
- Antipsychotics, antidepressants, and mood stabilizers used often to manage behavior
- Experimental therapies include vaccines, B-amyloid-protein breakers, and anti-t therapy (Bader & Littlejohns, 2004).

Nursing Interventions

- Caregiver support through individual and family counseling and support groups
- Education about disease process, comorbidities, and reasonable expectations for the future
- Educate on the importance of caregiver, self-care, and respite
- Environmental modifications such as calendars, clocks, pictures, safety locks, locked drawers and cabinets, and safe medication storage
- Behavior modification such as music therapy, crafts, and massage
- Maintain patient dignity and encourage activities to support quality of life
- Assist patients and families with execution of advanced directives
- Teach family and caregivers about behaviors (wandering, "sundowning," and agitation) and how to manage these challenging manifestations while maintaining safety
- Help families to identify that patient may be unaware of self-limitations (cooking, driving, and performing ADLs)
- Educate family and patient on slowed response to environmental cues
- Inform family/caregiver that patient can be easily distracted and cannot focus attention on current task (may forget about a pot of boiling water on the stove)
- Encourage family/caregivers to set boundaries with some limitations for ADLs, if unsafe
- Encourage ethical treatment of patient at all times
- Connect families to community resources such as adult day cares, respite, in-home personal aides, assisted living, and hospice
- Inform family about signs of disease progression that may lead to the need for total care
- Assist families in setting up daily routines that may benefit both parties
- Encourage families to advocate for loved ones by informing neighbors of the patient's potential to wander (Bader & Littlejohns, 2004)

Dystonia

Dystonia is a neurological syndrome manifested by involuntary sustained, patterned, and often repetitive contractions of opposing muscles that cause twisting movements or abnormal postures (Bader & Littlejohns, 2004).

Etiology

- Third most common movement disorder after Parkinson's disease and essential tremor
- 300,000 people affected in North America
- More common in Jews of Eastern European or Ashkenazi ancestry (Bader & Littlejohns, 2004)

Clinical Manifestations

- Repetitive movements
- Patterned movements (same group of muscles is repeatedly involved)
- Usually, exacerbation by voluntary motor activity
- Stress and fatigue can increase dystonic movements
- Associated tremor - relationship between dystonia and essential-type tremor (Bader & Littlejohns, 2004)

Classification

- By distribution
  - Focal - affecting a single body part
  - Cranial dystonia - blepharospasm, oromandibular dystonia, laryngeal dystonia, cervical dystonia (torticollis), limb dystonia (task-specific idiopathic such as "writer's dystonia"), leg dystonia, and truncal dystonia
  - Segmental dystonia - affects one or more contiguous body parts
  - Multifocal - affecting two or more contiguous parts of the body (cervical and leg dystonia)
  - Hemidystonia - unilateral dystonia
- By age
  - Generally, the earlier the onset of symptoms, the more likely the chance of progression with advancing age
- By etiology
  - Primary versus secondary - primary is an isolated neurological disorder; secondary results from other environmental variables (Bader & Littlejohns, 2004)

Pathophysiology

- Excessive co-contraction of antagonist muscles
- Overflow of contractions to adjacent or remote muscles

- Paradoxical contraction of passively shortened muscles (Bader & Littlejohns, 2004)

Differential Diagnosis

- Drug reactions
- Encephalitis
- Lesch-Nyhan (X-linked)
- DYTI (AD)
- Wilson's disease
- Mitochondrial disease
- Stroke
- Toxic cause (Hayden Gephart, 2013)

Treatment

- Botulinum injections - Clostridium botulinum (chemical denervation)
- Anticholinergics
- Benzodiazepines
- Anticonvulsants
- Lithium
- Reserpine
- Baclofen
- Levodopa (Hayden Gephart, 2013)
- Surgical
  - Selective peripheral degeneration
  - Lesioning surgery - includes deep brain stimulator (DBS) (Bader & Littlejohns, 2004)

Nursing Interventions

- Physical and occupational therapy
- Strengthen muscles that may be underused
- Promote optimal body posture
- Avoid sudden manipulations or extremes in movement (fight against the contractions)
- Provide supportive social treatment
- Encourage patient to express feelings
- Refer to support groups
- Instruct patient in stress management and relaxation
- Promote self-care activities
- Refer to community resources
- Educate patient and family about dystonia

Parkinson's Disease

Parkinson's disease (PD) is a neurodegenerative disease caused by a depletion of dopamine-producing cells in the substantia nigra. Cardinal features of PD include resting tremor, rigidity, bradykinesia, and diminished postural ability (Bader & Littlejohns, 2004).

Epidemiology

PD affects approximately 850,000 Americans, with 30,000 new diagnoses each year. This figure will rise as the baby boomer population ages. The annual financial burden of PD is estimated to be in excess of $5 billion. The greatest single risk factor for PD is advancing age. The incidence rate grows from 11 out of 100,000 in the general population to 50 out of 100,000 in those over 50 years of age. The median age of onset is 62 years of age. PD is rare below age 30, but 4-10% of cases occur before age 40. PD is slightly more common in men than in women.
- Rare below age 30
- 4-10% of cases by age 40
- Median onset is age 62
- Increased prevalence with age (Stacy, Davis, Heath, Isaacson, Tarsy, Williams, & Moore, 2013)

Pathophysiology

Neurodegeneration in PD is scattered in a multifocal distribution throughout the brain. This is a progressive process, presumably starting years or even decades before symptoms emerge and continuing over many years throughout the course of the disease. The motor features of the disease primarily result from loss of dopaminergic neurons of the substantia nigra that project to the caudate nucleus and putamen. Some motor and other non-motor features of the disease are likely due to loss of dopaminergic and non-dopaminergic innervation in other brain regions (Stacy, Davis, Heath, Isaacson, Tarsy, Williams, & Moore, 2013).

Etiology

- Primarily idiopathic (may involve mitochondrial dysfunction)
- No single causative agent has been identified in Parkinson's
- Genetic, environmental, cardiovascular, and secondary causes of PD have been postulated
- Occupational exposure to heavy metals, particularly copper and manganese, are associated
- Rural living has remained a prevalent risk factor in several research studies (exposure to pesticides and well water)
- Oxidative stress from free radicals that damage DNA (evident on postmortem brains) (Bader & Littlejohns, 2004)

Clinical Manifestations

- Classic triad-resting tremor, rigidity, and bradykinesia
- Postural instability - in late stages, patient has a stooped posture
- Retropulsion
- Falls
- Gait disturbance (shuffling, diminished arm swing)
- Dystonia
- Loss of dexterity
- Microphagia (handwriting samples are often small and illegible)
- Secondary manifestations - depression, dementia, anxiety, psychosis, apathy, and sleep disturbances (some dopamine agonists can cause daytime somnolence)
- Autonomic dysfunction - urinary incontinence, sexual dysfunction, constipation, orthostatic hypotension, impaired thermoregulation (hyperhidrosis), and sensory abnormalities
- Craniofacial abnormalities - dysphagia, blepharitis, dysarthria, and excessive drooling
- Seborrhea - seborrheic dermatitis is common in PD
- Weight loss
- Peripheral edema (Bader & Littlejohns, 2004)

Diagnosis

- History and physical
- Neuroimaging studies - very limited benefit because CT/MRI are basically normal
    o PET scan may show presynaptic nigral cell loss
    o SPECT - can show presynaptic dopaminergic deficits in patients
- Rating scales
    o Unified Parkinson's Disease Rating Scale (UPDRS) bedside evaluation tool that assesses:
        - Mentation, behavior, and mood
        - Activities of daily living
        - Motor examination
        - Complications of therapy
        - Modified Hoehn and Yahr staging
        - Schwab and England Activities of Daily Living Scale (Bader & Littlejohns, 2004)

Treatment

- Primarily dopamine agonism
- Levodopa (L-dopa) crosses into the CNS where it is converted into dopamine; Sinemet inhibits dopa decarboxylase to prevent metabolism of L-dopa
- COMT (catechol-O-Methyl Transferase) inhibitors to prevent the metabolism of L-Dopa
- Dopamine agonists (pergolide, bromocryptine)

- Monoamine oxidase inhibitors B (selegiline)
- Amantadine releases dopamine
- Anticholinergics (Benzhexol, benztropin (Cogentin), artane)
- Deep brain stimulation is used for patients with intolerable medication side effects (Hayden Gephart, 2013)

Caregiver and End-of-Life Issues

- Spouses are most often the primary caregiver for a person with PD. Caregiving in the later stages of the disease can present significant challenges and create substantial stress for caregivers.
- Multiple factors contribute to the stress of caregiving associated with PD:
  o Physical challenges
  o Transfers
  o Toileting
  o Bathing
  o Transportation
  o Emotional challenges
  o Change in marriage roles
  o Increased emotional needs of the caregiver, unmet by patient
  o Uncertainty about the future
  o Financial challenges
  o Unreimbursed medical costs
  o Loss of income from primary earner (Stacy, Davis, Heath, Isaacson, Tarsy, Williams, & Moore, 2013)

Nursing Care

- People with Parkinson's have specific needs and care requirements. Most important is that they receive their medication on time, every time. Nurses should also be aware of the "on/off" nature of the condition.
- Some patients say they are "on" when their drugs are working and symptoms are mostly under control. If they go "off," their symptoms are out of control, and it becomes harder for them to move; some may stop moving altogether. Patients might change from "on" to "off" very quickly like a switch.
- The way in which Parkinson's affects patients can vary from hour to hour and day to day, and it also varies widely between individual patients. The amount of help and support patients need also varies. Therefore, nurses should listen to patients and their families about how the condition affects them.
- It is important to ensure that patients have access to a varied and balanced diet; nurses should take account of any swallowing or movement problems that could lead to malnutrition. It is also important to remember to give patients time to answer when talking to them. It may take time for them to respond, but this does not mean they are not listening or do not understand.
- Nurses should act as advocates and participate in Advanced Care Planning with patients and families (Cotton, 2012).

Nursing Interventions

- Administer medications promptly on schedule to maintain continuous therapy drug levels.
- Encourage independence. Provide assistive devices as appropriate.
- Provide rest periods between activities.
- Provide frequent warm baths and massages to help relax muscles and relieve muscle cramps.
- Protect the patient from injury.
- Have the patient sit in an upright position when eating.
- Provide the patient with a semi-solid diet, which is easier to swallow than a diet consisting of solids and liquids.
- Monitor drug treatment and report any adverse reactions.
- Monitor for complications caused by involuntary movements such as aspiration or injury from falls.
- Evaluate the patient's nutritional intake and weigh him/her regularly (Bader & Littlejohns, 2004).

Peripheral Neuropathy

Peripheral neuropathy describes damage to the peripheral nervous system, which transmits information from the brain and spinal cord to every other part of the body. Peripheral neuropathy may be either inherited or acquired. Causes of acquired peripheral neuropathy include systemic disease, physical injury (trauma) to a nerve, tumors, toxins, autoimmune responses and disorders affecting nerve tissue, nutritional deficiencies, alcoholism, and vascular and metabolic disorders. Inherited forms of peripheral neuropathy are caused by inborn mistakes in the genetic code or by new genetic mutations (Neuropathy Association, 2013).

Etiology

Approximately 30% of neuropathies are "idiopathic," or of an unknown cause. In another 30% of cases, the cause is diabetes. Other neuropathy causes include autoimmune disorders, tumors, heredity, nutritional imbalances, infections, and toxins (Neuropathy Association, 2013).

Epidemiology

- Out of the 25 million people with diabetes mellitus in the U.S., 8% will experience neuropathy at the time of diagnosis.
- 50-60% of diabetics will experience neuropathy.
- Diabetes is associated with multiple neuropathies affecting the face, limb, and trunk (Bader & Littlejohns, 2004).

Etiology

- No hypothesis confirmed: theories are metabolic versus vascular
- Neuropathy is generally associated with other complications of DM.
- More likely in prolonged disease state; occurs mostly in tall males
- In type II DM, the association between hyperglycemia and neuropathy is not strong (Bader & Littlejohns, 2004).

Pathophysiology

- Unknown
- Axonal degeneration theory
- Microangiography theory (Bader & Littlejohns, 2004)

Prevention

- Tight glucose control (Bader & Littlejohns, 2004)

Assessment

- Subjective - pain, numbness, tingling, weakness
- Objective
  - Sensory loss in "stocking glove distribution"
  - Mild distal weakness may be present
  - Nerve conduction changes are the same in type 1 and type 2 DM
  - Nerve conduction changes are length-dependent
  - Sensory nerves are more likely to be affected
- Diagnostic - nerve conduction studies (Bader & Littlejohns, 2004)

Interventions

- Test serum glucose regularly
- Encourage patient to record blood sugars daily
- Medication to keep hemoglobin A1C within normal limits
- Assess skin, feet, and hands; intervene if necessary
- Educate about foot care and adapting to loss of sensation in the feet (Bader & Littlejohns, 2004)

Toxic Neuropathy

Toxic neuropathy involves painful paresthesias and dysesthesias in the limbs, usually distally. They are caused by a toxin, with or without weakness (Bader & Littlejohns, 2004).

Epidemiology

- Unknown

Etiology

- Occurs with accidental or intentional exposure to toxins
- Occurs after exposure to medications, particularly to certain antineoplastic agents
- Basic tenets
- Strong dose-response relationship
- Consistency of response at a specific dose
- Proximity of symptoms to exposure
- Improvement usually follows cessation of exposure
- Benign agent may enhance the toxicity of a known toxin that is present in safe levels (Bader & Littlejohns, 2004)

Classification

- Toxic materials
- Acrylamide - found in plumbing materials, textiles, packaging, and grout
- Arsenic - accidentally or intentionally placed in food (homicide/suicide)
- Hexacarbons - industrial material
- Lead - found in paint, moonshine, and bullets
- Mercury - thermometers, contaminated fish
- Organophosphates - used to kill parasites
- Thallium - Rodenticide (agent for homicide/suicide)
- Drugs - Platinum, chloramphenicol, cisplatin, colchicine, dapsone, disulfiram, amiodarone, gold, isoniazid, nitrofurantoin, pyridoxine (vitamin B6), Taxol, phenytoin, simvastatin, tacrolimus (FK506), thalidomide, vincristine, zalcitabine, and alcohol (Bader & Littlejohns, 2004)

Prevention

- Eliminate exposure to the toxin (Bader & Littlejohns, 2004)

Assessment

- Subjective - neuropathic pain, weakness, or both (other symptoms may be present depending on agent)
- Objective
  - Produces more motor than sensory signs in patients exposed to dapsone, disulfiram, nitrofurantoin, organophosphates, lead, vincristine
- Diagnostic
  - Identification of body burden (hair levels, blood and urine levels) often negative due to passage of time between exposure and diagnostic evaluation
  - EMG/NCV

- Quantitative sensory testing
- Identification of system involvement (Bader & Littlejohns, 2004)

Interventions

- Removal from the source of exposure
- Arsenic - Gastric lavage, Chelation with dimercaprol, D-penicillamine, or dimercaptosuccinic acid
- Inorganic lead - chelation with IV calcium disodium EDTA, oral dimercaoti-succunic acid, oral penicillamine
- Mercury - chelation with N-acetyl-D-penicillamine (Bader & Littlejohns, 2004)

Hereditary Neuropathy

- Charcot-Marie-Tooth (CMT) disease has several forms
  - All include pes cavus deformity of the feet, hammertoes, and distal weakness with atrophy of the extremities, primarily legs (Bader & Littlejohns, 2004)

Epidemiology

- Prevalence is 1 in 2,500 people (Bader & Littlejohns, 2004)

Etiology

- All cases are caused by mutations, which have been found on chromosomes 1, 8, 10, 17, and X. CMT is classified as CMT 1, CMT 2, CMT 4, or X-linked (Bader & Littlejohns, 2004).

Prevention

- Prevention is not possible because spontaneous mutations occur; genetic testing may be helpful (Bader & Littlejohns, 2004).

Pathophysiology

- All forms are characterized by demyelination or defective myelination. CMT 2 involves axonal loss in addition to abnormal myelin (Bader & Littlejohns, 2004).

Assessment

- Subjective
  - Feet deformities
  - Weakness in lower extremities and possibly hands
  - Family history
  - Sensory complaints or pain

- Objective
  - Deformity of feet including pes cavus and hammertoes
  - Distal weakness accompanied with atrophy in extremities; lower is usually more severe than upper
  - Reduced or absent DTRs
  - History of multiple compressive neuropathies
- Diagnostic
  - All except CMT 2 show slowing on nerve conduction velocity (NCV)
  - CMT 2 has normal NCV
  - Genetic testing (Bader & Littlejohns, 2004)

Potential Problems

- Risk for immobility
- Pain
- Contractures (Bader & Littlejohns, 2004)

Treatment

- Medical
  - Genetic testing
  - Counseling for patient and family
  - PT and OT (Bader & Littlejohns, 2004)

Nursing Interventions

- Assess and manage immobility and hazards
- Teach ROM exercises on unaffected limbs at least four times daily
- Position and alignment to prevent complications
- Provide progressive mobilization
- Link to resources and support groups
- Observe and teach the use of adaptive mobility and DME
- Acknowledge patient and family fears related to immobility and disability (Bader & Littlejohns, 2004)

Benign Essential Tremor

A benign essential tremor is the most common movement disorder of an unknown cause. A tremor is known as an oscillatory movement produced by alternating or synchronous contraction of opposing muscle groups. It typically involves a tremor of the finger, hands, or arms, but sometimes, involves the head or other body parts, during voluntary movements (Bader & Littlejohns, 2004).

Clinical Features

- Tremor, usually of hands and forearms, which is worsened by stress, anxiety, and movement
- Onset usually before age 30
- Improved with alcohol and propranolol (Bader & Littlejohns, 2004)

Pathophysiology

- Unknown, may involve increased activity of inferior olives (Bader & Littlejohns, 2004)

Etiology

- Usually associated with family history (Bader & Littlejohns, 2004)

Treatment

- Medical
  - Propranolol and primidone are first line
  - Benzodiazepines
- Surgical treatment
  - Thalamotomy or deep brain stimulation for severe patients (Bader & Littlejohns, 2004)

Degenerative Spine and Disc Disease

Spinal degeneration is a normal part of aging. Along with physiological changes, there can be associated symptoms that are problematic or disabling for patients.

- Physiological changes in both the composition and function of the disk
- Despite radiological indications, patients may be asymptomatic
- Symptoms include pain, dysfunction, and disability (Bader & Littlejohns, 2004)

Etiology

In a certain number of patients, disc degeneration leads to instability within the spine, and the spine is unable to bear the patient's weight or perform its normal functions without disabling pain (Bader & Littlejohns, 2004).

Symptoms

- Cervical disc degeneration can be characterized by neck pain. Often, the disc will be associated with osteophytes or bone spurs. They can further reduce movement and lead to nerve compression. The cervical nerve roots innervate the back of the head and neck as well as the arms and hands, and the patient can experience burning, tingling, numbness, and pain in these areas. Sometimes, headaches result from cervical disc degeneration.

- Lumbar disc degeneration is often associated with lower back pain. It is typically a weight-bearing type of back pain with severe pain when sitting. Prolonged periods of standing and walking can be painful, as can bending and lifting. Associated lumbar radiculopathy or nerve root pain may be accompanied by burning, numbness, tingling, and pain extending from the gluteus maximus and lumbar region down through the leg (Bader & Littlejohns, 2004).

Treatment

- Modification of body mechanics - avoidance of exacerbating movements like reclining or kneeling rather than sitting, not lifting in a bent position, and using a back brace are all options to try to reduce tensions and weight-bearing by the affected lumbar disc. The use of a cervical spine collar can facilitate this.

- Lifestyle modifications - patients who have degenerative discs in the lumbar spine may help with pain reduction by losing weight, building the back and stomach muscles through a fitness program, and exercising.

- Pain management - pain may be managed through working with a pain management specialist. Some therapies may include steroid injections, medication management, or a facet rhizotomy. This technique can achieve lasting pain relief for a year or more by ablation of the sensory nerve through the facet joint.

- Non-surgical treatment for degenerated lumbar discs is *intradiscal electrothermal annuloplasty* (IDET). This technique heats up discs proven to be painful by discography CT with a copper coil to a temperature that hardens the disc. It allows the disc to resist weight-bearing motion better than the degenerated disc in about 70% of patients.

- Surgical treatment - a spinal fusion can aid in the reduction or elimination of pain. It can be done from a posterior approach with screws and rods in the spine and adjacent bone graft or an anterior approach with removal of the disc and placement of graph materials in the front. Sometimes, surgeons will choose to place implants in the disc and the screws both from a posterior approach. With painful degenerative discs that cannot bear the patient's weight without severe pain, spinal fusion is highly successful in eliminating pain. If possible, surgery is generally avoided due to the acceleration of degeneration of adjacent discs (Bader & Littlejohns, 2004).

Vertebral Compression Fractures

Vertebral compression fractures occur as a result of bone weakened by osteoporosis, trauma, tumors, metastasis, or hemangioma. Osteoporosis accounts for a majority of vertebral fractures (Bader & Littlejohns, 2004).

Epidemiology

- Fracture occurs accompanied by loss of vertebral bone mass density due to the aging process
- Lifetime risk of an osteoporotic vertebral fracture in white females by age 80 is 50%
- Once a vertebral compression fracture occurs, the risk of additional fractures in adjacent vertebrae increases fivefold
- Compression fractures are present on radiograph at a rate of 500 per 100,000 people in patients 50-54 years old; 2,960 per 100,000 in people older than 85 years of age (Bader & Littlejohns, 2004)

Incidence

- Annual incidence of osteoporotic fractures is 260,000 in the U.S.
- Twice as common in females as in males, occurring in 153 per 100,000 females compared to 81 per 100,000 males (Bader & Littlejohns, 2004)

Etiology and Risk Factors

- Osteoporosis
- Advanced age
- Early/premature menopause and five years post-menopause without hormone replacement
- Medications associated with development of osteoporosis - steroids, anticonvulsants, cytotoxic therapy, excessive thyroxine, heparin, phenothiazines, and lithium
- ETOH, cigarette smoking, malnutrition, sedentary lifestyle, inadequate calcium intake, Caucasian race, and being underweight
- Metastatic disease of the spine
- Cancerous tumors may metastasize to the spine
- Vertebral hemangioma
- Trauma (Bader & Littlejohns, 2004)

Prevention

- Reduce risks of developing osteoporosis (early intervention and education in young women and men)
- Nutritional counseling
- Encourage exercise

- Smoking cessation
- Consider hormone replacement therapy, if not contraindicated
- Initiate aggressive treatment of osteopenia and osteoporosis (Fosamax, Evista, and calcium supplements) (Bader & Littlejohns, 2004)

Assessment

- Subjective
    - Sudden onset of back pain that may occur after a benign activity such as coughing or sneezing
    - Pain is often debilitating
    - Difficulty finding a comfortable position
    - Sleep difficulties related to pain
    - Pain is reproducible with manual palpation
    - Pain may be exacerbated by activity, sitting, or deep aspiration
- Objective
    - Myelopathy - neurological changes related to spinal cord compression
    - Lower spine weakness and paresthesias
    - Gait disturbances
    - Bowel/bladder dysfunction
    - Thoracic radicular pain characterized by sharp, stabbing, aching, or burning pain around the chest wall or rib in a dermatomal distribution
- Diagnostic
    - Plain spinal films - show fracture and alignment
    - CT scan
    - MRI - can assess neural compromise (Bader & Littlejohns, 2004)

Potential Problems

- Pain related to vertebral displacement (Bader & Littlejohns, 2004)

Treatment

- Medical
    - Rest during acute symptoms
    - Early mobilization
    - Analgesics - narcotics, acetaminophen, and NSAIDs
    - Muscle relaxants in short-term
    - Gabapentin (Neuromuscular) or tricyclic antidepressants for radicular pain
    - Local application of heat/ice
    - Orthotics - bracing may improve pain and reduce deformity; TLSO (thoracolumbosacral orthosis), Jewett hyperextension brace, or corset
- Surgical
    - Indicated to decompress the spinal cord if there is posterior displacement of bone or retropulsion of bone fragment into the spinal canal; if there is no compression, the patient may be a candidate for vertebroplasty or kyphoplasty

- Vertebroplasty - radiological procedure that treats intense pain associated with vertebral compression fractures
  - Indicated in patients whose pain remains severe and debilitating and refractory to maximal medical treatment
  - Inclusion criteria - pain localized to a fracture or tumor, pain refractory to medical management, fracture <12 months old, patient must be able to lie prone for the entire procedure
  - Exclusion criteria - fracture that extends to posterior vertebral cortex; retropulsed fragment in the spinal canal; spinal cord compression, radiculopathy, osteomyelitis, or diskitis; fever or sepsis; coagulopathy
  - Involves injection of acrylic cement (polymethylmethacrylate) into collapsed vertebral body
  - Does not restore height of the vertebral body
- Kyphoplasty - refinement of the vertebral procedure
  - Relieves pain and restores some or all of the vertebral height
  - Indicated for treatment of acute vertebral fracture secondary to osteoporosis or trauma
  - Injection of methylmethacrylate is a thicker consistency than that used in vertebroplasty
- Nursing interventions
  - Vertebroplasty
    - Acute care: patient must lie flat for one to two hours before sitting and walking with assistance; may be discharged once stable with non-narcotic medications and muscle relaxants
    - Post-hospitalization/recovery phase: encourage patient to remain as active as possible; educate that pain may persist for a few days
  - Kyphoplasty
    - Acute care: patient must lie flat for one to two hours before sitting and walking with assistance; if stable, discharge with muscle relaxant and non-narcotic medication (acetaminophen and/or NSAID); encourage patient to remain as active as possible; instruct patient that pain may persist for a few days post-procedure
  - Lifestyle modifications – nutrition, exercise, smoking cessation, body mechanics, weight loss
  - Medications
    - Educate patients on Fosamax, Actonel, Miacalcin, calcium; vitamin D and vitamin C supplements; and hormone replacement therapy
    - Review medication regimen and identify any medications that may predispose to osteoporosis
- Diagnostics
  - Serial testing of bone density with dual-energy x-ray absorptiometric (DEXA) scans (Bader & Littlejohns, 2004)

Lumbar Spondylolisthesis

Degenerative spondylolisthesis (DS) is a disorder that causes the slip of one vertebral body over the one below it due to degenerative changes in the spine (Kalichman & Hunter, 2007).

Epidemiology

- Lumbar spondylosis is present in 27-37% of the asymptomatic population
- In the U.S., more than 80% of individuals older than 40 years of age have lumbar spondylosis, increasing from 3% of individuals 20-29 years of age (Kalichman & Hunter, 2007)

Etiology

- Lumbar DS is a major cause of spinal canal stenosis and is often related to lower back and leg pain
- Appears to be a non-specific aging phenomenon

Pathophysiology

- Lumbar spondylosis occurs as a result of new bone formation in areas where the annular ligament is stressed (Kalichman & Hunter, 2007).

Assessment

- Subjective
    - Common complaint of patients with DS is back pain
    - Patients usually report that their symptoms vary as a function of mechanical loads (such as in going from supine to erect position) imposed, and pain frequently worsens over the course of the day (Kalichman & Hunter, 2007)
- Objective
    - The most probable sources for signs and symptoms related to DS are: 1) degenerated and subluxated facet joints; 2) segmental instability that cause tension of facet joint capsule and ligaments as well as overuse of stabilization muscles; and 3) spinal stenosis and intervertebral foramen stenosis
    - Pain that has been episodic and recurrent for many years
    - Radiation into the posterolateral thighs is also common and is independent of neurologic signs and symptoms
    - The pain may be diffuse in the lower extremities, involving the L5 and/or L4 roots unilaterally or bilaterally
    - Leg pain that shifts from side to side
    - Symptoms of neurogenic claudication
        - Pain in lower back and leg
        - Pins and needles going down leg
        - Weakness

- Bowel or bladder problems may occur if the neurogenic claudication is severe
- Relieved by stooping, bending, or sitting (Kalichman & Hunter, 2007)
- Diagnostic
  - Plain films
  - CT
  - Myelography
  - contrast material-enhanced CT
  - MRI (Kalichman & Hunter, 2007)

Treatment

- Use of analgesics and NSAIDs to control pain
- Epidural steroid injections
- Physical methods such as bracing and flexion-strengthening exercises
  - PT, rehabilitation, chiropractic care
- Surgery (criteria)
  - Non-operative treatment is first line
  - Persistent or recurrent back and/or leg pain or neurogenic claudication with significant reduction of quality of life despite a reasonable trial of non-operative treatment (minimum of three months)
  - Progressive neurological deficit
  - Bladder or bowel symptoms (Kalichman & Hunter, 2007)

Prognosis

- Favorable
- Only 10-15% of patients seeking treatment will eventually have surgery
- 76% of patients without neurological deficits at initial examination remained without neurological deficits after 10 years of follow-up (Kalichman & Hunter, 2007)

Lumbar Spinal Stenosis

Lumbar spinal stenosis is a disorder that is characterized by any narrowing of the lumbar spinal canal, lateral recess, or neural foramina. It can be congenital or acquired. A patient may have significant stenosis or may be asymptomatic with a lesser degree of stenosis (Bader & Littlejohns, 2004).

Epidemiology

- Symptoms usually affect men 50 years of age or older
- Male to female ratio is 8:1 for bilateral lower extremity symptoms
- Male to female ratio is 3:1 for unilateral lower extremity symptoms (Bader & Littlejohns, 2004)

Etiology

- Central canal stenosis
  - Narrowing of the lumbar spinal canal
  - This compresses the thecal sac and thus, the cauda equina
  - Neurogenic claudication (lower extremity pain, paresthesia, heaviness, or weakness that spreads from the legs to the buttocks and lower back when walking)
    - Relieved when person sits back down (Bader & Littlejohns, 2004)

Pathophysiology

- Neurogenic claudication or intermittent claudication
  - Compressive theory: compression of the spinal nerve roots
  - Ischemia theory: insufficient blood flow to the nerve roots during walking
  - Stagnant anoxia theory: stagnation of blood flow and CSF
  - Likely related to inadequate oxygenation or accumulation of metabolites in the cauda equina
  - Nerve function may be adequate at rest and inadequate during exercise (Bader & Littlejohns, 2004)

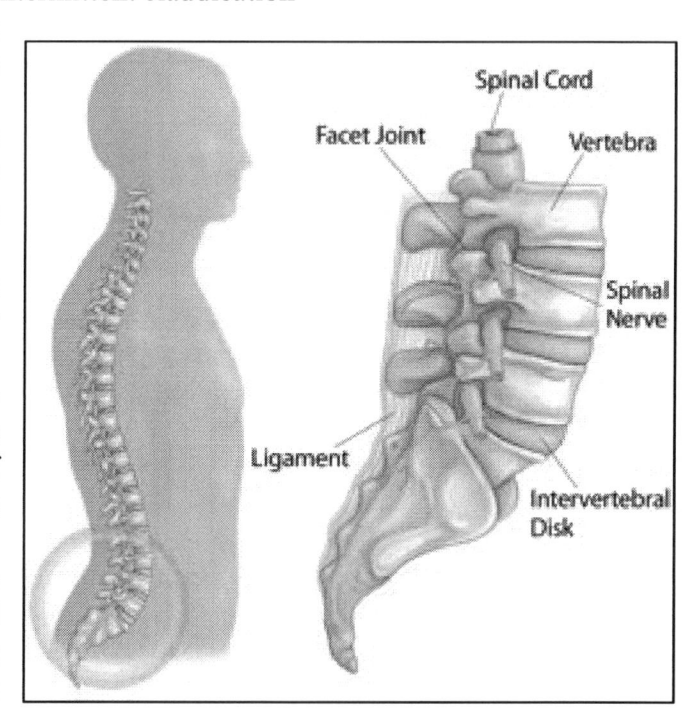

Assessment

- Subjective
  - Pain with ambulation leading to gradual decrease in ambulation
  - Able to ambulate farther if using a grocery cart or other assistive device for forward flexion support
  - May complain of bowel and bladder dysfunction
- Objective
  - Strength is generally normal, but can have bilateral deficits or multilevel deficits with severe stenosis
  - Reflexes may be diminished or absent due to nerve compression; if hyperreflexic, needs further workup; sensation may be normal

- o Stance/gait may be stooped; known as "Simian" stance
- o With comorbidities like diabetes, may have "stocking" decrease in sensation, indicative of peripheral neuropathy
- Diagnostic
    - o Lumbar spine/AP/lateral plain film - evaluate alignment
    - o Myelogram/CT - evaluates bony structure better than MRI
    - o Electromyography/nerve conduction (EMG/NCS)
    - o Vascular testing if insufficiency is suspected (Bader & Littlejohns, 2004)

Interventions

- Medical
    - o PT; epidural steroid injections; nerve root blocks (Bader & Littlejohns, 2004)
- Surgical
    - o Total laminectomy with foraminotomy; single or multilevel
        - Decompress the thecal sac and cauda equina
    - o Bilateral laminotomy
        - Preserves central ligamentous structure
    - o Unilateral approach for bilateral decompression
        - Less post-operative pain
    - o Fusion
        - Indicated if there is spinal instability (Bader & Littlejohns, 2004)
- Nursing care
    - o Acute care
        - Monitor VS as per post-operative policy
        - Monitor neurological function
            - o Residual lower extremity symptoms are common in the initial post-op period
        - Administer pain medication as prescribed and document response
        - Observe surgical dressing for bleeding or drainage (Bader & Littlejohns, 2004)
    - o Rehabilitation
        - Patients requiring surgical intervention have become quite sedentary due to symptomatology
        - Patient may benefit from short inpatient rehab stay if deconditioned (Bader & Littlejohns, 2004)
    - o Post-hospitalization/recovery phase
        - Should avoid stretching exercises, bending, lifting, and twisting for the first four to six weeks for muscular healing
        - Can gradually increase ambulation, progressively increasing strength and endurance
        - Outpatient PT may be beneficial (Bader & Littlejohns, 2004)

Craniosynostosis

Craniosynostosis is a birth defect that causes premature closure of one or more sutures of the skull (Bader & Littlejohns, 2004).

Epidemiology

- Occurs in 1 of every 2,100 births
- Classifications
    o Sagittal synostosis accounts for 40-60% of cases
    o Coronal synostosis accounts for 20-30% of cases
    o Metopic synostosis accounts for 10% of cases
    o Lambdoid synostosis occurs in <3 out of 100,000 (Bader & Littlejohns, 2004)

Etiology

- Position in utero and genetics affect craniosynostosis
- The earlier the closure, the more severe the deformity (Bader & Littlejohns, 2004)

Pathophysiology

- Neurocranium is composed of vault of skull (calvaria) and cranial base
    o Calvaria is formed from intramembranous bone of paraxial mesodermal and neural crest origin (desmocranium)
    o Ossification of calvarial bones depends on the presence of brain (anencephaly is absence of brain, which results in calvaria)
    o Frontal, parietal, and occipital bones form calvaria
    o Bones are separated by sutures
        - Sagittal: suture between parietal bones
        - Metopic: suture between frontal bones
        - Coronal: suture between frontal and parietal bones
        - Lambdoid: sutures between occipital and parietal bones (Bader & Littlejohns, 2004)
    o At birth, the neurocranium has achieved 25% of ultimate growth
        - Half growth occurs at six months of age
        - By 2 years of age, 75% of growth has occurred
        - By 10 years of age, 95% of growth has occurred
    o Growing brain exerts tension on bone, thus stimulating sutural bone growth
        - Head circumference is a good indicator of brain growth (Bader & Littlejohns, 2004)

Assessment

- Sagittal suture synostosis
    o Subjective: parents report unexplained irritability and fussiness before surgical release of suture and a decrease in these behaviors immediately afterward

- o Objective: elongated head, frontal bossing, bitemporal narrowing, occipital cupping, and palpable bony ridge along sagittal suture line
- o Diagnostic: made by physical examination, skull films (AP/Lateral), and CT scan
- Coronal suture synostosis
  - o Subjective: some parents report unexplained irritability and fussiness before surgical release of suture and a decrease in these behaviors immediately afterward
  - o Objective: eye on affected side pulled upward; harlequin sign on AP skull film; forehead flattened on affected side; nasal root deviated to affected side, making nose appear "twisted"
  - o Diagnostic: made by physical examination, skull films (AP/Lateral), and CT scan
- Metopic suture synostosis
  - o Subjective: some parents report unexplained irritability and fussiness before surgical release of suture and a decrease in these behaviors immediately afterward
  - o Objective: sutures start to close by the second year (this is the only suture that completely disappears); patient has *hypotelorism* (closed-set eyes)
  - o Diagnostic: made by physical examination, skull films (AP/Lateral), and CT scan
- Lambdoid suture synostosis
  - o Subjective: some parents report unexplained irritability and fussiness before surgical release of suture and a decrease in these behaviors immediately afterward
  - o Objective: occipitoparietal flattening, palpable bony ridge over lambdoid suture, bony prominence at skull base behind ear on affected side; skull has a trapezoid shape when viewed from above
  - o Diagnostic: made by physical examination, skull films (AP/Lateral), and CT scan (Bader & Littlejohns, 2004)

Interventions

- Potential concerns: children with misshapen heads may be ridiculed among peers because they are different; may not be able to wear hats or pull shirt over heads; may have increased ICP, which lowers IQ
- Surgical
  - o Traditional approach consists of "pi procedure," calvarial vault remodeling, wide vertex craniotomy, partial morcelization, strip craniectomy, lateral canthal advancement, orbitofrontal bandeau advancement and strip craniectomy, partial or complete occipital bone reconstruction
  - o Endoscopic strip craniectomy - less invasive than traditional approach and 1/4 of the cost; less blood loss and shorter inpatient stay (overnight)
  - o Custom-made modeling helmet is worn for approximately one year to reshape the skull

Nursing Interventions

- Teach post-op care, hospital stay, and expected outcomes (normocephaly)
- Refer patients with coronal synostosis to pediatric ophthalmologist
- Assess pain using age-appropriate pain scale
- Reassure parents and let them stay with their child to provide comfort
- Asses VS, labs, color, activity level, and signs & symptoms of bleeding
- After endoscopic strip craniectomy, a baby with sagittal synostosis should lie with the back of his/her head on a mattress until the helmet is worn to decrease AP distance
- A helmet mold is constructed three to four days after surgery for endoscopic strip craniectomy
- Helmet adjustments and/or remolding are completed four to six weeks post-op and every three months after one year (Bader & Littlejohns, 2004)

Meniere's Disease

Meniere's disease is a disorder of the inner ear. It can cause severe dizziness, a roaring sound in your ears called tinnitus, hearing loss that comes and goes, and the feeling of ear pressure or pain. It usually affects only one ear. It is a common cause of hearing loss (Bader & Littlejohns, 2004).

Friedrich's Ataxia

- A progressive, hereditary spinocerebellar disorder
- Onset between 8 and 15 years of age
- Slow degenerative changes in the spinal cord and brain that affect speech and motor coordination and produce numbness and weakness of the limbs, lower limb paralysis, and areflexia
- Occurs in 1 out of 40,000 people
- Individuals eventually become dependent for most ADLs
- Life span is 35-40 years of age
- Death is related to cardiac complications or respiratory compromise
- Result of mitochondrial iron accumulation leading to cellular damage and death by free radical toxicity
- Gait worsening in the dark is reported
- Cardinal features: gait and limb ataxia, absent lower limb reflexes, extensor plantar responses, dysarthria, and reduction or loss of vibration sense and proprioception
- Genetic testing can diagnose
- Nerve conduction studies: absent sensory nerve action potentials and reduced motor nerve conduction velocities
- ECG and ECHO: evidence of cardiomyopathy
- Loss of somatosensory EPs and auditory brainstem responses (Bader & Littlejohns, 2004)

Trigeminal Neuralgia

- Description
    - Trigeminal neuralgia (TN) is a painful facial condition of unknown etiology
    - One of the most common causes of facial pain
    - It was originally known as tic douloureux (tic)
    - Also termed idiopathic and primary trigeminal neuralgia (Wood, 2004)

Symptoms

- The primary symptom of TN is pain of a neuropathic nature with both chronic and acute elements
- The clinical hallmark is a sudden, excruciating, repetitive attack of unilateral facial pain (known as a paroxysm) in the distribution of one or more branches of the trigeminal nerve
- It is often precipitated by trivial mechanical stimulation such as touching, eating, washing, shaving, brushing the teeth, or talking
- The condition is chronic, and over time, the pain intensifies, episodes become longer and more frequent, and the pain spreads to larger areas of the face (Wood, 2004).

Epidemiology

- The trigeminal nerve, or fifth cranial nerve, emerges from the base of the brain (pons) and possesses both sensory and motor fibers.
- It is one of the largest nerves in the head and has three main branches, which are distributed to different areas of the face, and is responsible for sending the impulses of touch, pain, pressure, and temperature from the different areas of the face to the brain (National Institute of Neurological Disorders and Stroke, 2013).
- The paroxysm of pain usually occurs unilaterally, most commonly on the right-hand side of the face, although, in 3-4% of patients, it can occur on both sides simultaneously.
- The pain is usually localized along the maxillary or mandibular branch, or both, and is occasionally felt along the ophthalmic branch.
- It is estimated that the prevalence of TN is 1 per 1,000 people, with an average age of onset of 50 years.
- The condition appears to be more common in women, and incidence increases with age.

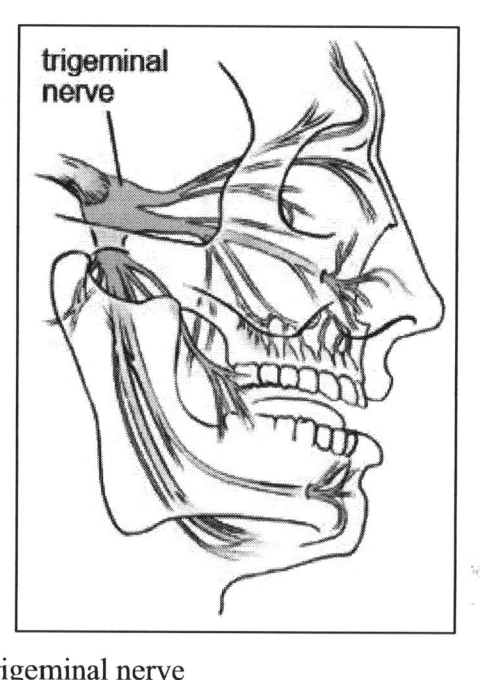

- There are few epidemiological studies of TN, and its long-term prognosis, impact on psychological well-being, morbidity, and comorbidity for patients is therefore largely unknown (National Institute of Neurological Disorders and Stroke, 2013).

Etiology and Pathophysiology

- The etiology and pathophysiology of TN remain unknown. It is hypothesized that the pain is caused by compression of the trigeminal nerve at its entry into the pons, which leads to demyelination—the loss of the myelin sheath. In turn, demyelination results in the transmission of abnormal pain messages, subjecting the patient to neuropathic pain.
- Compression of the trigeminal nerve can be due to a number of factors including tumor (10% of patients), pressure from blood vessels, aneurysm, and multiple sclerosis; causes of damage to the myelin sheath include nerve injury, shingles or post-herpetic neuralgia, trauma, infection, degeneration of the teeth or jaw, and the aging process.
- If the patient has a lesion, multiple sclerosis, or other conditions that can cause neuropathic pain in the trigeminal nerve, the TN is said to be secondary or symptomatic rather than primary or idiopathic (Wood, 2004).

Contributing Factors

- Multiple sclerosis
- Non-smoker
- Non-alcohol user
- Hypertension
- Not having undergone tonsillectomy
- Familial clustering, although reports for this are contradictory (Wood, 2004)

Assessment and Diagnosis

- There are no objective measures, such as laboratory or pathological tests, available to diagnose TN, and physical and neurological examinations and investigations often yield normal results.
- However, some can be helpful in establishing whether the TN is idiopathic or secondary and/or determining the extent and location of any nerve compression.
- Diagnostic
    - CT
    - MRI
    - MRA
    - The International Headache Society suggests that these clinical criteria be present before making a diagnosis of TN:
        - The pain of TN occurs in paroxysms, which can last from several seconds to two minutes and can vary in frequency from several hundred a day to periods of remission lasting weeks or years.

- - Typically, the pain is sudden in onset, severe in degree, and short in duration. Patients use terms such as "sharp," "stabbing," "burning," "shooting," and "like an electric shock" to characterize the pain and describe it as "unbearable," "terrible," "excruciating," and "intense." The pain is so severe that it causes patients to wince, which is why TN is also known as a tic. As time progresses, the paroxysms can become more frequent and severe.
    - Patients tend to be asymptomatic between the paroxysms and are generally pain-free at night. However, some experience a background pain that is dull, aching, and continuous.
  - The McGill Pain Questionnaire is suggested as an assessment tool for TN, as it has been shown to differentiate between TN pain and atypical facial pain and also to assess pain intensity and quality and psychological distress.
  - A pain diary can also be used to assess the frequency and severity of attacks, to assess the ability of the patient to perform normal activities, and to monitor the response to treatments and any adverse reactions (Wood, 2004).

Management and Treatment

- Medical management remains the first-line treatment for most patients, but if this fails to control the pain or if intolerable side effects occur, surgical management must be considered.
- Anticonvulsants
  - Anticonvulsant drugs are effective in reducing TN pain for many patients.
  - Their mechanism of action remains unclear, but it has been proposed that they decrease pain impulses and produce pain relief by:
    - Blocking sodium channels
    - Acting as antagonists on the N-methyl-D-aspartate (NMDA) mechanism
    - Suppressing the release of glutamate
    - Before carbamazepine therapy is initiated, full blood count and liver function tests should be performed
      - Decreased platelets or white blood cells may occasionally be associated with carbamazepine use, and patients should be asked to report any fever, sore throat, rash, ulcers in the mouth, easy bruising, and petechial or purpuric hemorrhages.
      - Careful control and monitoring is necessary, especially in older patients.
      - The drug should be started in low doses and increased, following a graduated protocol, until pain has been relieved.
      - If relief has not been achieved after six to eight weeks, carbamazepine should be discontinued.
    - Phenytoin is often a second-line therapy if carbamazepine is ineffective or if the patient cannot tolerate an effective dose
      - It is associated with additional side effects of carbamazepine, and there is no evidence to support its long-term use to treat TN

- o Phenytoin has been replaced with lamotrigine and gabapentin in clinical practice
  - Lamotrigine is used as an adjunct to carbamazepine for TN and has been found to be effective with few side effects.
    - o It can also be used as a monotherapy to treat mild pain.
  - Gabapentin is used for pain and has been shown to be an effective treatment for other neuropathic pains.
    - o The main advantage of gabapentin is its relatively benign side effects, which are usually well-tolerated if doses are increased gradually, following a graduated protocol.
- o Other drugs
  - Baclofen is used effectively in some patients, either as an adjunct to carbamazepine or as a monotherapy, although there is insufficient evidence for its use in TN.
    - o It is not licensed for use in TN, but has fewer side effects than carbamazepine.
  - If carbamazepine cannot be tolerated or is ineffective or if the patient is awaiting neurosurgery, tricyclic antidepressants (TCA) such as amitriptyline can be used.
    - o The side effects of amitriptyline, which include dry mouth, constipation, blurred vision, tachycardia, urinary hesitancy, orthostatic hypotension, dizziness, and tachycardia, can be minimized by slow titration of the dosage.
  - Topically administered capsaicin has also been used.
    - o Its side effects include transient burning and erythema, and it initially causes a burning sensation followed by anesthesia.
    - o The cream must be applied three to five times per day, which may negatively affect compliance.
  - Other drugs sometimes used with the drugs mentioned above include mexiletine, clonazepam, local anesthetics, non-steroidal anti-inflammatory drugs, and opioids (Wood, 2004).
- Surgical intervention
  - o If medical intervention is ineffective or cannot be tolerated by the patient, there are a number of surgical options available.
  - o There is currently no definitive evidence on when surgery should be considered.
  - o Surgical intervention can be focused for three levels: peripheral nerve branches, gasserian ganglion, and posterior fossa
    - Cryotherapy, laser treatments, injections, neurectomy, microcompression, radiofrequency coagulation, and microvascular decompression (MVD)
    - Only MVD causes no destruction of the trigeminal nerve (Wood, 2004)
- Other interventions
  - o The management of TN requires a multidisciplinary approach; however, there is little to no evidence to support their use. Some patients report that other treatment options offer some form of relief: acupuncture, distraction

techniques, relaxation training, biofeedback, meditation, and physical therapy (Wood, 2004).

Nursing Interventions/Considerations

- The nurse's role in assessing and managing patient pain is vital and will vary enormously depending on the setting.
- In the case of patients with TN, their pain is likely to be managed primarily through a specialist unit or pain service, which is multidisciplinary.
- Therefore, the nurse is usually a specialist or consultant nurse and will have additional skills to be able to assess and manage pain of a complex nature.
- The specialist nurse role will vary from service to service, but may include specialist assessment techniques, advising on pharmacological interventions and reviews, offering a variety of psychological and physical therapies, and being an educator.
- The role will involve liaising with other health professionals and services.
- Patients will be cared for in the community by a nurse, whose main role will be assessing and ensuring that any changes in the pain are managed appropriately and, when necessary, seeking specialist advice.
- Nurses in acute care settings must ensure that appropriate assessment of patient pain is undertaken and, when necessary, ensure that referrals are made (Wood, 2004).

Chapter 7: Sleep Disorders

Sleep and wake are alternating behavioral states over the course of a 24-hour day. Behaviorally, sleep is known as the temporary disengagement from and unresponsiveness to environmental surroundings. Also, sleep is a necessary process for restorative physiological function (Redeker & McEnany, 2011).

Typical Sleep Behaviors

- Closed eyes
- Little movement
- Recumbent posturing
- Reduced responsiveness to stimulation (Redeker & McEnany, 2011)

Stages of Sleep

The stages of sleep are based on brain wave activity, eye movements, and muscle tone.
- Sleep is divided into two distinct stages:
    - Non-rapid eye movement (NREM)
        - NREM sleep is divided into three stages (N1, N2, and N3)
            - An individual usually spends only a few minutes in stage N1, followed by stage N2 sleep.
            - Stage N2 is characterized by specific types of EEG waveforms called sleep spindles (12 and 14 Hz) and K complexes (large, slow waves of <1 Hz)
            - Most of a night of sleep is spent in stage N2.
            - Stage N3 follows stage N2 and is often called slow-wave sleep (SWS)
    - Rapid eye movement (REM)
        - Follows NREM sleep; is characterized by episodic bursts of rapid side to side eye movements, postural muscle atonia, and low-amplitude EEG patterns that resemble waking
        - Occurs in discrete times of night
        - Associated with vivid dreaming
        - Declines with age
- One complete sleep cycle includes an episode of NREM sleep followed by an episode of REM sleep
    - The average healthy adult will go through four to six cycles of 60-110 minutes (Redeker & McEnany, 2011).

Insomnia

Insomnia is defined as a complaint of disturbed sleep in the presence of an adequate opportunity and circumstance for sleep. The complaint may consist of difficulty initiating sleep, difficulty maintaining sleep, waking up too early, or non-restorative or poor-quality sleep. The diagnosis is made when the difficulty with sleep has a negative effect on daily function (Bloom, 2009).

Primary insomnia implies that no other cause of sleep disturbance has been identified. Comorbid insomnia is more common and is most often associated with psychiatric disorders (depression, anxiety, or substance use), medical disorders (cardiopulmonary disorders, neurological disorders, or chronic somatic complaints), medications, and other primary sleep disorders (OSA or restless legs). Comorbid insomnia does not suggest that other conditions "cause" insomnia, but rather that insomnia and the other conditions co-occur and that each may warrant clinical attention and treatment. Diagnosis of insomnia requires that an individual have difficulty falling and staying asleep for at least one month and that the effects have a negative influence on daytime functioning (Bloom, 2009).

Obstructive Sleep Apnea (OSA)

- Common symptoms of sleep apnea are loud snoring, choking or gasping episodes during sleep, and excessive daytime sleepiness that the patient may attribute to poor sleep.
- Insomnia is not a common complaint in patients with obstructive sleep apnea. However, if the suspicion of sleep apnea is high, the patient should be further investigated (Centers for Sleep, 2007).

Periodic Limb Movements in Sleep (PLMS)

- PLMS can occur at any age, but are more common in people over 45 years of age.
- Although these limb movements are often associated with brief arousals, many patients have no sleep complaints or daytime impairment.
- When these limb movements are associated with insomnia or daytime sleepiness, periodic limb movement disorder may be diagnosed (Centers for Sleep, 2007).

Restless Legs Syndrome (RLS)

- Patients with restless legs syndrome experience a difficult to describe, uncomfortable sensation of the limbs that comes on at rest and is relieved by movement such as walking.
- This restlessness occurs during a waking state and causes a delay in sleep onset.
- Periodic limb movement disorder commonly co-exists with restless legs syndrome.
- Iron deficiency, renal failure, pregnancy, and SSRI antidepressants are commonly associated with restless legs syndrome (Centers for Sleep, 2007).

Circadian Rhythm Disorders

- Delayed and advanced sleep phase, shift work sleep disorder, and jet lag are the most common circadian rhythm sleep disorders.
- Delayed sleep phase (DSP) results in difficulty falling asleep at a normal time and waking up in the morning.

- These disorders commonly occur in teenagers and can significantly distress the individual and his/her parents.
- Advanced sleep phase (ASP) occurs in the elderly and is associated with an abnormally early bedtime and difficulty with early morning awakening.
- Adolescents tend to have a natural sleep phase delay, so there is a greater biologic tendency to be a "night owl" during puberty.
- Behavioral issues (computer gaming, instant messaging, listening to music, etc.) can certainly worsen this transient predisposition.
- The elderly tend to have a natural sleep phase advance, so there is a tendency to become a "lark" with advancing age.
- Jet lag and shift work sleep disorders are complex, multi-factorial problems.
- Effective management of circadian rhythm sleep disorders is achieved through behavioral strategies, light therapy, and appropriate use of melatonin (Centers for Sleep, 2007).

Secondary/Co-Morbid Insomnia

- Psychiatric disorders
  - Approximately 40% of outpatients who complain of insomnia have it on the basis of a psychiatric disorder
  - Psychiatric disorders are most commonly associated with co-morbid insomnia
  - The relationship is poorly understood and is likely "bi-directional;" therefore, the clinician should not expect that management of the psychiatric illness will resolve the insomnia
  - The NIH consensus document emphasizes the importance of treating insomnia independently in patients suffering from psychiatric illness
  - A significant body of literature has examined the sleep disturbance of patients with major depression
    - Antidepressants (SSRIs and SNRIs) used to treat such patients may have a direct effect on the sleep pattern
    - One condition that can be exacerbated by SSRI and SNRI antidepressants is restless legs syndrome
    - These medications are known to increase motor activity during sleep, and this effect can last up to one year after discontinuation of treatment (Centers for Sleep, 2007).
- Medical disorders
  - Many medical conditions disrupt sleep through a variety of mechanisms. Some of the common conditions that cause secondary insomnia are:
    - Chronic Pain Syndromes
    - Menopause
    - Gastroesophageal Reflux and Peptic Ulcer Disease
    - COPD/Asthma
    - Benign Prostatic Hyperplasia (Centers for Sleep, 2007)

- Medications
  - Alerting or stimulating drugs taken late in the day will often contribute to poor sleep. Examples include:
    - Nicotine, nicotine patches
    - Caffeine, caffeine-containing medications (e.g. Anacin)
    - Antidepressants (SSRIs, SNRIs, bupropion, opiates)
    - Corticosteroids
    - Central nervous system stimulants and related drugs
      - Dextroamphetamine
      - Methylphenidate
      - Atomoxetine
      - Bronchodilators
      - Pseudoephedrine (Centers for Sleep, 2007)

Other Considerations

- Alcohol and stimulants such as nicotine and caffeine may cause poor sleep
  - While consumption of alcohol before bedtime promotes sleep onset, alcohol tends to shorten total sleep time and can exacerbate other conditions such as gastroesophageal reflux and sleep apnea.
  - Alcohol withdrawal in a heavy drinker may be associated with restlessness or tremor
  - Objective alterations in sleep architecture have been observed in alcoholics following 12 months of abstinence
- Diagnosis and management of the primary sleep disorder and/or secondary cause of the insomnia is critical to the overall management of the patient complaining of insomnia.
  - Primary insomnia that occurs subsequent to and associated with a primary sleep disorder or co-morbidly with a medical or psychiatric disorder is difficult to manage (Centers for Sleep, 2007).

Medications Used to Treat Sleep Disorders

- Amitriptyline (Elavil and others)
- Amoxapine (Asendin and others)
- Bupropion (Wellbutrin), buspirone (BuSpar)
- Carbidopa-levodopa (Sinemet and others)
- Citalopram (Celexa), clonazepam (Klonopin and others)
- Clorazepate (Tranxene and others)
- Desipramine (Norpramin and others)
- Desmopressin (DDAVP and others)
- Dextroamphetamine (Dexedrine and others)
- Diazepam (Valium and others)
- Doxepin (Sinequan and others)
- Estazolam (ProSom and others)

- Fluoxetine (Prozac)
- Flurazepam (Dalmane and others)
- Fluvoxamine (Luvox)
- Medroxyprogesterone (Provera and others)
- Methylphenidate (Ritalin and others)
- Mirtazapine (Remeron)
- Modafinil (Provigil)
- Nefazodone (Serzone)
- Nortriptyline (Pamelor and others)
- Paroxetine (Paxil)
- Pemoline (Cylert)
- Pergolide (Permax)
- Phenelzine (Nardil)
- Phenobarbital (Donnatal and others)
- Pramipexole (Mirapex)
- Protriptyline (Vivactil)
- Ropinirole (Requip)
- Selegiline (Eldepryl)
- Sertraline (Zoloft)
- Temazepam (Restoril and others)
- Tranylcypromine (Parnate)
- Trazodone (Desyrel and others)
- Triazolam (Halcion and others)
- Trimipramine (Surmontil)
- Venlafaxine (Effexor)
- Zaleplon (Sonata)
- Zolpidem (Ambien) (Pagel & Parnes, 2001)

Nursing Interventions

- Assess for signs and symptoms of a sleep pattern disturbance such as statements of difficulty falling asleep or not feeling well-rested as well as interrupted sleep, irritability, disorientation, lethargy, frequent yawning, or dark circles under eyes.
- Determine the client's usual sleep habits
- Perform actions to reduce fear and anxiety
- Discourage long periods of sleep during the day unless signs and symptoms of sleep deprivation exist or if daytime sleep is usual for client
- Perform actions to relieve discomfort, if present (e.g. reposition client; administer prescribed analgesics, antiemetics, or muscle relaxants)
- Encourage participation in relaxing diversional activities during the evening
- Discourage intake of foods and fluids high in caffeine (chocolate, coffee, tea, colas) in the evening
- Unless contraindicated, offer client an evening snack that includes milk or cheese (the L-tryptophan in milk and cheese helps induce and maintain sleep)

- Whenever possible, allow client to continue usual sleep practices (position; time; and pre-sleep routines such as reading, watching television, listening to music, and meditating)
- Before sleep, satisfy basic needs such as comfort and warmth
- Encourage client to urinate just before bedtime
- Reduce environmental distractions such as closing door to client's room, using night light rather than overhead light whenever possible, lowering volume of paging system, keeping staff conversations at low level and away from client's room, closing curtains between clients in a semi-private room or ward, and keeping beepers and alarms on low volume
- Provide client with "white noise" such as a fan, soft music, or tape-recorded sounds of the ocean or rain
- Have sleep mask and earplugs available for client, if needed
- Ensure good room ventilation
- Encourage client to avoid drinking alcohol in the evening (alcohol interferes with REM sleep)
- Encourage client to avoid smoking before bedtime (nicotine is a stimulant)
- If possible, administer medications that can interfere with sleep (e.g. steroids and diuretics) early in the day rather than in late afternoon or evening
- Administer prescribed sedative-hypnotics, if indicated
- Perform actions to reduce interruptions during sleep (80-100 minutes of uninterrupted sleep is usually needed to complete one sleep cycle)
- Restrict visitors
- Whenever possible, provide group care (e.g. medications, treatments, physical care, and assessments)
- Consult appropriate healthcare provider if signs and symptoms of sleep deprivation persist or worsen (Redeker & McEnany, 2011)

Chapter 8: Toxic Encephalopathies

- The term "toxic encephalopathy" is used to indicate brain dysfunction caused by toxic exposure.
- Chronic toxic encephalopathy, cerebellar syndrome, Parkinsonism, and vascular encephalopathy are commonly encountered clinical syndromes of toxic encephalopathy.
- The signs and symptoms of toxic encephalopathy may be mimicked by many psychiatric, metabolic, inflammatory, neoplastic, and degenerative diseases of the nervous system (Kim & Kim, 2012).

Epidemiology

- According to the U.S. Environmental Protection Agency, more than 65,000 commercial chemicals are currently used in the U.S., and 2,000-3,000 new chemicals are added to this list each year.
- The number of neurotoxic chemicals currently used in industry is unknown, but an unadventurous estimate might suggest more than 1,000.
- People may be exposed to these neurotoxins due to their occupations, occasionally at home, or through other inadvertent mechanisms (Kim & Kim, 2012).

Etiology

- The CNS is protected from toxic exposure to some extent, but it remains vulnerable to the effects of certain chemicals found in the environment.
- Non-polar, lipid-soluble substances (e.g. organic solvents) gain the easiest access to the CNS, where neurons are particularly susceptible due to their high lipid contents and metabolic rates. Both gray matter and white matter can be easily damaged by lipophilic toxins (Kim & Kim, 2012).

Pathophysiology

- Dose-response relationship in the majority of toxic encephalopathies
- Typically manifests as a non-focal or symmetrical neurological syndrome
- Strong temporal relationship between exposure and symptom onset
- The nervous system has a limited capability to regenerate compared to other organs such as the liver or hematopoietic system. Thus, more sequelae persist after the removal of a neurotoxic agent compared to toxic diseases of other organs.
- Multiple neurological syndromes may occur in response to a single neurotoxin, depending on the level and duration of the exposure.
- Clinical disorders of the CNS have varying presentations, often involving a host of non-specific symptoms. Furthermore, few neurotoxins cause patients to present with a pathognomonic neurological syndrome.

- Asymptomatic toxic encephalopathy may be seen in occupational or environmental settings.
- The timing of exposure relative to critical periods of CNS development may explain some of the variations in susceptibility.
- Neurotoxins may reduce the functional reserves of the brain, potentially making the cells more vulnerable to the effects of aging and leading to accelerated senescence (Kim & Kim, 2012).

Clinical Syndromes of Toxic Encephalopathy

- Acute diffuse toxic encephalopathy
    - Reflects a global cerebral dysfunction of rapid onset (typically days or weeks) and may be associated with alterations in the level of consciousness
    - Causative agents include organic solvents, which can alter cellular membrane function, and some gases (e.g. gas anesthetics, carbon monoxide, hydrogen sulfide, and cyanide), which can diffusely affect brain function
    - Heavy metals can also cause acute encephalopathies; this is more commonly associated with organic metals (e.g. methyl mercury, tetraethyl lead, and organic tin) than with inorganic metals (e.g. mercury, lead, and tin)
    - Clinical manifestations, which depend on the neurotoxin and intensity of exposure, can range from mild euphoria with a normal examination to stupor, seizure, coma, and even death
    - Diagnosis does not generally present a challenge for acute syndromes because exposure and clinical manifestations are likely to be closely linked in time
    - In patients with severe acute toxic encephalopathy, an MRI of the brain may show focal areas, most commonly bilateral basal ganglia, or diffuse areas of edema.
    - Treatment of diffuse acute encephalopathy is primarily supportive, starting with removal of the exposure source.
    - For most of the neurotoxins that act diffusely on the brain, recovery from acute exposure is complete (Kim & Kim, 2012).

- Chronic toxic encephalopathy (CTE)
    - CTE usually represents a chronic persistent diffuse injury to the brain resulting from cumulative or repeated exposures (often over a period of months or years) to solvents or (occasionally) heavy metals
    - Clinical manifestations of CTE usually involve varying degrees of cognitive impairment
    - CTE is an established, internationally recognized condition that results from excessive occupational exposure to solvents via inhalation or skin contact
    - The severity of CTE is graded as I to III or 1, 2A, 2B, and 3
    - Type I CTE and types 1 and 2A CTE include subjective symptoms relating to memory, concentration, and mood
        - At this stage, clinicians may miss the diagnosis by considering these symptoms as a psychiatric issue due to altered mood

- Type II CTE and type 2B CTE are characterized by objective evidence of attention and memory deficits, decreased psychomotor function, and/or learning deficits in neurobehavioral testing
- Detailed occupational and medical histories, as well as standardized neurobehavioral testing, are the cornerstones of the standard diagnostic process.
- The diagnosis of CTE requires a careful clinical assessment that 1) establishes that there is evidence for abnormality, mainly in neuropsychological testing; 2) determines that there is good evidence of exposure to a potentially hazardous neurotoxin; and 3) excludes any other underlying causes.
- Specific therapies for CTE are limited. The patient should be separated from the neurotoxic exposure as soon as possible. Once the toxin has been removed, the reversibility of the brain damage will depend on the grade of CTE (Kim & Kim, 2012).

- Cerebellar syndromes
    - Gait ataxia, dysarthria, intention tremor, gaze-evoked nystagmus, dysmetria, and adiadochokinesia can all result from cerebellar dysfunction
    - Neurotoxin-induced cerebellar syndrome, which is a clinical entity that can be differentiated from solvent-induced CTE or carbon-disulfide-induced vascular encephalopathy, is sometimes accompanied by other neurological findings
    - If a patient presents with cerebellar dysfunction, a detailed history of his/her occupation and neurotoxin exposure should be obtained
    - Methyl mercury intoxication (Minamata disease)
    - Methyl bromide intoxication - inhalation
    - Organic tin intoxication (Kim & Kim, 2012)

- Parkinsonism
    - Manganese intoxication (manganism)
    - Manganism is one of the most typical forms of Parkinsonism.
    - Chronic excessive exposure to manganese can affect the globus pallidus, resulting in parkinsonian signs and symptoms, sometimes along with psychiatric features such as locura manganica or manganese madness.
    - Historically, miners developed psychosis due to exposure to manganese at levels of up to several hundred milligrams per cubic meter.
    - The clinical course of manganism can be divided into three stages:
        - First stage: patients with manganism usually have prodromal neuropsychiatric symptoms such as asthenia, apathy, somnolence, irritability, emotional lability, or frank psychoses.
        - Second stage: bradykinetic-rigid parkinsonian syndrome with dystonia, which is reversible, presents as the main clinical feature.
        - Last stage is notable for aggravation of the signs and symptoms described above. In some cases, the clinical progression has been found to be irreversible and persistent after the cessation of exposure.
    - Therefore, early diagnosis of manganism is important (Kim & Kim, 2012).

- Vascular encephalopathy
  - Carbon disulfide poisoning is a highly typical and frequently encountered vascular encephalopathy
  - Patients with carbon disulfide poisoning exhibit various clinical characteristics including multiple brain infarctions, peripheral neuropathy, coronary heart disease, retinopathy (including microaneurysm of the fundus), hypertension, glomerulosclerosis of the kidney, and parkinsonian symptoms.
  - These findings indicate that the basic mechanisms underlying carbon disulfide poisoning involve atherosclerotic changes in blood vessels.
  - The clinical manifestations of vascular encephalopathy (e.g. hemiparesis and speech disturbance) in cases of chronic carbon disulfide poisoning are similar to those observed in patients with atherosclerotic cerebrovascular disorders.
  - Many patients presenting with acute cerebrovascular stroke-like symptoms, sometimes with hypertension or diabetes, have been misdiagnosed as having suffered cerebrovascular attacks.
  - Thus, the possibility of carbon disulfide poisoning must not be overlooked when physicians make differential diagnoses in patients with vascular encephalopathy (Kim & Kim, 2012).

- Neurodegenerative diseases
  - Amyotrophic lateral sclerosis (ALS)
  - ALS is a neurodegenerative disease with an annual worldwide incidence of 2-4 cases per 100,000 individuals.
  - The association between ALS and exposure to solvents or lead is unclear, and even the best-designed incidence studies have produced conflicting results (Kim & Kim, 2012).

- Other neurodegenerative diseases
  - It is reported that exposure to solvents, aluminum, mercury, or pesticides is implicated in the development of Alzheimer's disease, which is the most common neurodegenerative disease (Kim & Kim, 2012).

Diagnostic Approaches for Toxic Encephalopathy

- A diagnosis of toxic encephalopathy can be made after documentation of the following: 1) a sufficiently intense or prolonged exposure to the neurotoxin; 2) a neurological syndrome appropriate for the putative neurotoxins; 3) evolution of signs and symptoms over a compatible temporal course; and 4) exclusion of other neurological disorders that may account for a similar syndrome (Kim & Kim, 2012).
- Exposure history, physical examination, neurological examination, and additional laboratory and radiological studies are particularly important for diagnosing a toxic encephalopathy (Kim & Kim, 2012).
- Acquisition of a detailed exposure history
  - The patient's exposure history is central to an accurate clinical diagnosis.
  - Exposure data such as workplace airborne concentrations are crucial.

- o A detailed evaluation of the nature, duration, and intensity of the exposure is essential for every evaluation.
- o A description of the availability and use of personal protective equipment will provide further information about the extent of possible exposure.
- o It is also important to ask questions about hobbies, and inadvertent exposure from any source should be considered.
- o For the diagnosis of toxic encephalopathy, it is likely to be helpful if information on similar problems observed in others at the worksite is available (Kim & Kim, 2012).
- Neurological examination
  - o Non-neurological signs may be a clue to toxic exposure; examples of systemic clues include blue gums in lead intoxication, Mees' lines in arsenic poisoning, and acrodynia in mercury poisoning.
  - o The neurological examination will generally assess mental function (mental status examination), cranial nerve function, muscle strength and tone, reflexes (muscle stretch and cutaneous stimulation), sensation, station, and gait.
  - o A complete and rigorous neurological examination is necessary to properly define the clinical neurological syndrome involved (Kim & Kim, 2012).
- Clinical laboratories
  - o When a patient is seen close to the time of exposure, it may be possible to measure the offending chemical, such as lead and mercury, or its metabolite in blood or urine.
  - o Biomarkers can demonstrate exposure to the relevant toxin and whether the exposure was sufficiently severe to give rise to a clinical syndrome.
  - o Occasionally, there may be paraclinical features in hematological and biochemical tests indicating red blood cell changes such as in lead poisoning or liver function test abnormalities such as in some organic solvent poisoning.
  - o For most neurotoxins, however, clinical laboratory tests are not helpful for diagnosis (Kim & Kim, 2012).
- Neurobehavioral testing
  - o Neurobehavioral (neuropsychological) testing, which is an accepted methodology for assessing the functional integrity of the CNS, has been used extensively to evaluate subclinical neurotoxic effects on cognition, memory, alertness, executive function, mood, and psychomotor function (Kim & Kim, 2012).
- Electroencephalography (EEG)
  - o EEG, which records the electric activity of the brain, has been used to evaluate occupational neurotoxic exposures.
  - o The most obvious changes on an EEG, such as diffuse slowing, are often associated with toxic encephalopathy (Kim & Kim, 2012).
- Evoked potentials (EVPs)
  - o Sensory EVPs are widely used in clinical neurology as an index of the integrity of the sensory CNS pathways.
  - o EVPs can provide more quantitative information and can be used to assess a sensory pathway from the receptor to the cortex (Kim & Kim, 2012).

- Neuroimaging
    - Neuroimaging can be divided into two groups: morphological neuroimaging (anatomy-based imaging) such as CT and MRI; and functional neuroimaging (physiology-based imaging) such as magnetic resonance spectroscopy (MRS), functional MRI, diffusion tensor imaging (DTI), SPECT, and PET (Kim & Kim, 2012).

Treatment

- Hyperbaric oxygen therapy (HBOT) has been shown to reduce ischemia and its damage in a wide range of tissues including, but not limited to, the nervous system.
- Increased lipid peroxides are present in the majority of toxic injury patients.
- HBOT reduces lipid peroxides; it also facilitates healing of damaged nerves in the brain as well as in the peripheral nervous system.
- Increased formation of lipid peroxides occurs with toxic injury (directly through detoxification changes with increased free radical production and indirectly through inflammation) (Kim & Kim, 2012).

Delirium

- Also referred to as "altered confusional state" (ACS)
- ACS is characterized by abrupt onset of behavioral change and short duration (hours to weeks; rarely months).
- Major characteristic of altered attention behaviors
    - DSM-IV (1994) criteria
        - Clinical features that develop over a short period of time and tend to fluctuate
        - Reduced clarity of awareness of the environment, disturbance of attention, or both
        - At least two of the following: perceptual disturbance, incoherence of speech, disturbance of sleep-wake cycle, and change in psychomotor activity
            - Disorientation, memory impairment, or both
            - Evidence of a specific organic factor judged to be etiologically related
        - The key difference between ACS and long-term psychiatric conditions is the acute onset (Bader & Littlejohns, 2004).

Etiology/Contributing Factors

- Precipitating illnesses: systemic illnesses (CV events, infections, fever, metabolic problems)
- Drug intoxication with psychoactive sedative-hypnotics, barbiturates, antidepressants, neuroleptics, narcotics, alcohol
    - Abrupt withdrawal of drug or abrupt initiation of drugs commonly used in acute care

- Metabolic and nutritional imbalances
- Neurological disorders: chronic subdural hematomas undiagnosed at time of hip fracture
- Iatrogenic disorders of hospitalization: anesthesia, MI, CHF, respiratory failure, sensory overload and deprivation (ICU delirium)
- Mnemonic for reversible causes of confusion: MIND ESCAPE
    - Metabolic/biochemical abnormality
    - Infection/impaction/inability to void/injury
    - Neoplasm/nutritional deficiency/normal pressure hydrocephalus
    - Drug withdrawal
    - Environmental toxins/environmental changes
    - Sleep deprivation, sensory overload/sensory deprivation
    - Cardiac/cerebrovascular/CND disease
    - Alcohol/alcohol withdrawal/anemia
    - Pain
    - Emotional/mental illness (Bader & Littlejohns, 2004)

Assessment/Treatment

- Most important is to suspect ACS with changes in behavior; consider behavior before the illness (history and family input important); pre-existing emotional/psychiatric disease, conditions, cognitive delusions or behavior that appear commonly at waking or falling asleep (Bader & Littlejohns, 2004)
- Treatment: first order is to begin treatment for reversible causes and etiologies
    - Pharmacological: small doses of antipsychotics and antidepressants are used
        - Useful for extreme fear states, delusion, and hallucinations
        - Start slowly, go slowly, and discontinue as soon as possible
        - In elderly, treatment of underlying cause may lag due to liver and kidney function (Bader & Littlejohns, 2004).
    - Non-pharmacological
        - Provide reassurance
        - Ordered environment and decreased stimulation for agitation
        - Increased stimulation and attention for lethargy
        - Diversional activities are useful for long-term ACS patient
        - Families encouraged to help maintain reality of patient and abate fear of common harm (Bader & Littlejohns, 2004)
    - Restraint use and misuse
        - Use of restraints is controversial and has legal implications in agitated and confused/delirious states
        - General rule is to use the least restrictive environment
        - Restrained patients require more supervision
        - Restraints can increase fear
        - Side rails are now considered a restraint - high risk for injury (Bader & Littlejohns, 2004)

Chapter 9: Pain

- Pain can be described as an unpleasant sensory and emotional experience associated with either actual or potential tissue damage.
- An individualistic, physiologic, learned, and social response to a noxious stimuli
- Always subjective; the source is difficult to identify, and the intensity is difficult to quantify (Bader & Littlejohns, 2004)
- *Acute*
    - Thought to be a warning signal to the body that something is wrong or needs attention
    - Signs and symptoms include: patient self-report, tachycardia, hypertension, tachypnea, shallow respirations, agitation or restlessness, facial grimace, splinting, and hypotension as a sign of patient-related shock.
    - Objective signs and associated autonomic nervous system hyperactivity with tachycardia, hypertension, and diaphoresis are present.
    - Duration is of recent onset, 0 to 70 days, and lasts <6 months.
    - Patients usually give a clear description of its location, character, and timing, leading to an etiological diagnosis.
    - The setting of the pain, its meaning, and its duration all influence the patient's ability to tolerate it.
    - Acute pain is usually self-limiting (Bader & Littlejohns, 2004).
- *Chronic*
    - Best described as the persistence of pain for ≥ three months
    - Pain that persists a month longer than the usual course of acute pain
    - May be associated with a chronic pathological process that causes continuous pain, or the pain recurs for months or years
    - Can lead to significant changes in a person's lifestyle, personality, and functional ability, compromising the patient's quality of life
    - Baseline pain refers to the average pain intensity expressed for 12 hours or more in a 24-hour period
    - Causes are not life-threatening
    - Treatment focuses on pain reduction, and adjuvants are primarily used (Bader & Littlejohns, 2004).

Epidemiology

- 70-90% of patients with advanced cancer report pain.
- 50% of cancer pain and surgical pain is unrelieved.
- Leads to lost time at work and decreased enjoyment in life and may lead to chronic pain
- Of nursing home patients that reported cancer-related pain, 24% received nothing more than aspirin.
- At least 40 million Americans suffer from chronic headaches and spend $40 billion per year on medications (Bader & Littlejohns, 2004).

Etiology and Contributing Factors

- Causes
    - Injury/trauma
    - Demyelinating disease
    - Metabolic disease
    - Infection
    - Neoplasm
    - Nerve injury
    - Vascular disease
    - Post-therapeutic neuralgia
    - Diabetic neuropathy
    - Complex regional pain syndrome
    - Phantom limb pain
    - Trigeminal neuralgia
    - Intervertebral disc disease/spinal stenosis with root compression
    - Compression of plexus
    - Entrapment syndromes
    - Inflammation
    - Neoplasia
    - Headache
- Genetic predisposition - familial history with headache, neuropathic pain, and diabetic neuropathy
- Theories of pain
    - Pain is emotion
    - Pain has two parts - sensation and reaction
    - Specificity theory - pain is related to specific anatomic structures and physiological functions
    - Pattern theory - articulated to account for the abnormal pain states not explained by the specificity theory (phantom pain)
    - Gate control theory - a complex perceptual experience influenced by physiological factors unique to the individual
    - Psychological theories of pain
        - Pain is an emotion or the manifestation of an emotional state; dates back more than two millennia to Aristotle
        - Pain perception and tolerance relate to prior experiences including social modeling, culture, attentional focus, suggestions by others, anxiety, and perceived meaning or cause of pain.
        - Behavioral theories of pain, like Pavlov's, believe in cognitive reward for pain relief (Bader & Littlejohns, 2004).

Pathophysiology

- Pain pathway
    - Nociceptive pain (related to stimuli from somatic and visceral structures)

- o Spinal cord modulation (received response from visceral and somatic nociceptive fibers)
- o Neurotransmitter modulation (tachykinins and dynorphin are excitatory; inhibitory modulators GABA, enkephalins, serotonin, 5-htp, norepinephrine, and adenosine receptors)
- o Ascending pathways
  - Spinothalamic tract: most important pain path in brain
  - Spinoreticular tract: produces arousal associated with pain perception
  - Spinomesencephalic tract: projects to midbrain and reticular formation
  - Spinocervical tract
  - Dorsal columns (Bader & Littlejohns, 2004)

Assessment

- Subjective
  - o Patient self-report; diary; verbal report
  - o Comprehensive history and physical
  - o Initial pain assessment tools/instruments
    - PQRST: provocative and palliative factors; quality of pain, radiation of pain, severity of pain, and timing of pain
    - OLDCART: O = onset; L = location; D = duration; C = characteristics; A = aggravating factors; R = relieving factors; T = treatment
    - ABCDE: acronym for pain assessment and management
    - Pain inventory: focus is on pain over the past 24 hours
    - Visual analog scale (VAS)
    - Verbal rating scale (VRS): uses adjectives that describe different intensities
    - Pain distress scale (0-10)
    - Picture of faces scale: good to use in pediatrics and with those with low literacy rate
    - Conditions and age-related considerations
      - o Tools include: FLACC, neonatal pain assessment scale (NPAS), CHEOPS, Wong-Baker FACES pain rating scale
      - o Elderly patients: assessment may be complicated by poor memory, depression, and sensory impairment
      - o Cognitively impaired patients: individualized assessments; behavioral indicators may be limited due to disease process
    - Hints to evaluating pain
      - o Be consistent with assessment tool
      - o Documentation related to treatment should be clear and describe effects of treatment
      - o Patient and family education/teaching
      - o Professional misconceptions must be addressed
      - o Regular communication with patient, family, and entire team
      - o Communication should focus on the goal of pain management and should include functional effects of pain and pain relief

- o Usage of pain diary
    - Evaluation of OTC drug use and other chemicals for pain relief
        - o Herbals, drugs, nicotine, alcohol
    - Psychosocial evaluation
        - o Consider effects of pain on life
        - o Psychiatric interview may be necessary to assess coping and mental health issues
        - o Use psychometric/pain-related techniques; Beck Depression Inventory, Sickness impact profile, McGill Pain Questionnaire
    - Diagnostic tests
        - o Labs: C-reactive protein, sedimentation rate, drug levels
        - o Radiological evaluation to rule out anatomic pathology: CT, MRI, plain X-ray films
        - o Electromyography and nerve conduction velocity (Bader & Littlejohns, 2004)

Treatment

- Pharmacological management
    - o Guidelines for implementation - use analgesia with the least side effects to determine the type of pain and pain source adjuncts
        - If patient is pain-free for months, consider a slow taper
        - Use multiple disciplines and non-pharmacological strategies
        - Adjuvant medications - administer antidepressants or anticonvulsants that are also analgesic for some painful conditions
            - o Adjuvant analgesics - no one mechanism of action for pain relief can be identified for this analgesic group; mild to moderate pain; inhibit the release of prostaglandin and thromboxane 2
        - Analgesics
            - o Non-opioids (acetaminophen, NSAIDs) - Prostaglandin, an anti-inflammatory mediator, is released when cells are damaged. Non-opioids sensitize nerves that carry information about pain.
            - o Opioids - these relieve pain mainly by action within the CNS, binding to opioid receptor sites in the brain and spinal cord.
                - Full agonist and pure agonist (morphine-like drugs)
                - Codeine, morphine, hydromorphone, and propoxyphene
                - All types of pain respond to opiates
                - When a drug attaches to opioid receptor sites as an antagonist, pain relief and other effects are blocked (naloxone)
                - Hydromorphone: five to six times more potent than morphine
            - o Anticonvulsants
            - o Corticosteroids
            - o Antiarrhythmics (sodium channel blocker)
            - o Antidepressants
            - o GABA B agonists
            - o Anti-epileptics

- Topical agents (Bader & Littlejohns, 2004)
- Routes
  - Parenteral: continuous, patient-controlled analgesia; via central or peripheral venous access; CNS side effects such as sedation or respiratory depression may easily occur with patient who is narcotic-naïve
    - Overdosage - prevent by teaching the patient, who may be using a PCA, to report excessive sedation, and teach what the expected outcomes are in terms of pain intensity
  - Subcutaneous (SC) - used when patient is intolerant to oral pain medications or if IV vascular access is not desirable or available; morphine is commonly used
  - Intraspinal opioid analgesia - epidural and intrathecal space
    - Preservative-free hydrophilic opioids (Duramorph) are the first-line opioids for intraspinal route
  - Local anesthetics - administering local anesthetics affects the outside of the spinal cord; doses are reduced
    - Bupivacaine is used mostly
    - Fewer opioid side effects
    - Side effects are postural hypotension, which is treated with IV fluids, and numbness at the desired dermatome level
  - Implanted (intraspinal) infusion - pumps can continuously infuse concentrated medication into an intrathecal or epidural space
    - Can administer opioids, local anesthetics, a GABA agonist, and baclofen
  - Peripheral nerve and spinal cord stimulation - involves the use of electrical stimulation along a nerve using varying pulse width and amplitudes to decrease pain
    - Reported to be effective in 53-70% of patients
- Physical modalities
  - Stimulation techniques have good effect on steady pain; spinal cord-TENS, acupuncture, massage, exercise, thermotherapy, cryotherapy, and pressure
  - Physical, occupational, and behavioral therapy - education, consultation, and referral
- Psychosocial interventions
  - Relaxation, meditation, and imagery; biofeedback; cognitive distraction and reframing; patient education; psychotherapy and structured support; and support groups and pastoral counseling
- Invasive interventions
  - Non-neuroablative point injections - for trigger points
  - Intra-articular injections - steroid injections in between joints
  - Intercostal block - injection in between the intercostal spaces
  - Epidural steroid injection
  - Sympathetic blocks (Bader & Littlejohns, 2004)

Nursing Considerations

- Teach about medication including dosage and side effects
- Teach pre-operative/pre-procedure processes before surgery
- Educate about the pain management plan
- Monitor and document on flow sheet whether IV or intraspinal route
- Monitor respiratory rate for one full minute for accuracy - determine quality; if it drops below 8 to 10 breaths/minute or becomes shallow with poor quality and/or if the patient becomes difficult to arouse, stop opioid immediately
- Administer naloxone every two to five minutes as necessary for a maximum dose of 10 mg (Bader & Littlejohns, 2004)

Chapter 10: Chemical Dependency

Chemical dependency, substance abuse, addiction – the destructive use of psychoactive substances has many names, and nurses in any specialty will care for patients who are impacted by such issues. Chemical dependency is defined as compulsive drug use despite the negative consequences (Harvard University, 2004).

Statistics on Chemical Dependency

- The White House Office of National Drug Control Policy conducted a survey and found that between 1988 and 1995, Americans spent over $57 billion on illegal drugs.
- The Lewin Group for the National Institute on Drug Abuse found that in 1992, the estimated total economic cost of alcohol and drug abuse was $245.7 billion. This estimate included costs for substance abuse treatment, costs associated with decreased work productivity and lost job time, costs associated with drug-related crime, and expenditures for social welfare programs.
- The Drug Abuse Warning Network (DAWN) estimated that in 2005, there were 816,696 emergency department visits associated with illicit drug use, 492,655 emergency department visits associated with alcohol use, and 598,542 emergency department visits associated with non-medical use of prescription drugs.
- According to the Centers for Disease Control and Prevention, the rates of morbidity and mortality related to alcohol abuse are enormous. It has been estimated that each year, there are over 100,000 deaths caused by alcohol, making it the third leading cause of preventable mortality
- According to the Centers for Disease Control and Prevention, cigarette smoking is responsible for approximately 438,000 deaths in the U.S. each year.
- The 1996 National Household Survey on Drug Abuse estimated that there are 13 million users of illicit drugs in the U.S., that 10% of Americans abuse or are dependent on alcohol, and that 25% of Americans smoke.
- The 2002 National Survey on Drug Use and Health found that approximately 46% of all Americans – 108 million people – had tried an illicit drug at least once in their lives.
- Deaths from overdose have increased by 540% since 1980 (Harvard University, 2004).

Pathophysiology

- Reward pathway
  - When a human being or other animal performs an action that satisfies a need or fulfills a desire, the neurotransmitter dopamine is released into the nucleus accumbens and produces pleasure. It signals that the action promotes survival or reproduction, either directly or indirectly.
  - Addictive drugs provide a shortcut. Each in its own way sets in motion a biological process that results in flooding the nucleus accumbens with

dopamine. The pleasure is not serving survival or reproduction, and evolution has not provided our brains with an easy way to withstand the onslaught.
- After repeated use, cell receptors within the nucleus accumbens shut down, and larger amounts of the substance are needed to produce the same effect (Harvard University, 2004).

Diagnostic Criteria

The Diagnostic and Statistical Manual (DSM) is the diagnostic classification system for psychiatric disorders that was developed by the American Psychiatric Association. According to the DSM, a person can be considered dependent if three or more of the following behaviors are present:
- Tolerance to a psychoactive substance
- Withdrawal signs and symptoms when the substance is withheld
- The substance is often taken in larger amounts or over a longer period of time than was intended
- Unsuccessful efforts, or a persistent desire, to cut down or control substance use
- A great deal of time is spent in activities necessary to obtain the substance or recover from its effects
- Important social, occupational, or recreational activities are given up or reduced because of substance use
- Continued substance use despite knowledge of persistent or recurring physical or psychological problems likely to be caused or exacerbated by the substance ("Chemical Dependency")

Etiology and Contributing Factors

- Genetics
  - Research on families has shown that children of alcoholics are at a three to fourfold risk for developing alcoholism, and studies of twins appear to support a genetic basis for alcoholism
- Socio-cultural influences
  - Especially in large urban areas
- Psychological influences
  - History of sexual and/or physical abuse
  - Early onset of experimentation with psychoactive drugs
  - Low self-esteem
  - A propensity for risk-taking behavior
  - Impulsivity
  - Antisocial behavior
  - Male gender
  - Mental disorders such as schizophrenia, attention deficit hyperactivity disorder, depression, anxiety, obsessive compulsive disorder, and bipolar disorder
  - Perfectionism
  - Inability to delay gratification ("Chemical Dependency")

Drugs of Abuse

- Can be legal or illicit (illegal) substances (tobacco, alcohol)
  - Alcohol - most commonly abused substance
    - Increases the effects of the inhibitory neurotransmitter *gamma aminobutyric acid* (GABA) at GABA receptors and inhibits the effect of the excitatory neurotransmitter *glutamate* at N-methyl-d-aspartate (NDMA) receptors
    - Alcohol intoxication is marked by slurred speech, incoordination, impaired judgment, and decreased inhibitions.
    - In large doses, it is a central nervous system and respiratory system depressant, and it causes hypotension.
    - Long-term use is associated with liver disease, heart failure, brain atrophy, gastritis and ulcers, anemia, and various cancers; it is particularly dangerous to unborn children ("Chemical Dependency")
  - Amphetamines (meth, speed)
    - Act by directly stimulating the adrenergic nerve endings and causing a release into the synapses of norepinephrine and dopamine, neurotransmitters that stimulate the peripheral α receptors and β receptors
    - Acute intoxication causes anxiety, diaphoresis, tachycardia, and hypertension
    - More serious effects are seizures, hallucinations, psychosis, dysrhythmias, myocardial ischemia, hyperthermia, and rhabdomyolysis
    - Long-term effects include vasculitis, cardiomyopathy, pulmonary hypertension, aortic and mitral regurgitation, and permanent damage to the dopaminergic and serotonergic neurons ("Chemical Dependency")
  - Cocaine (white powder, crack)
    - Cocaine has many complex actions, but its effect can best be defined as a hyperadrenergic state that occurs through its effect on the neurotransmitters epinephrine and norepinephrine.
    - Acute intoxication from cocaine produces euphoria, agitation, tachycardia, hypertension, and increased respiratory rate.
    - It can also produce an enormous list of serious medical complications such as stroke, myocardial infarction, bowel infarction, aortic dissection, arrhythmias, hyperthermia, rhabdomyolysis, and pneumothorax.
    - Long-term effects of cocaine abuse include cardiomyopathy; increased atherosclerosis; left ventricular hypertrophy; endocarditis; impotency; hypertension; weight loss; malnutrition; and behavior that can be characterized as virtually identical to personality disturbances, paranoia, and schizophrenic syndromes ("Chemical Dependency")
  - Heroin (smack)
    - Heroin acts by stimulating opioid receptors in the brain. When these receptors are stimulated, the cells become hyperpolarized (thus becoming less active and less able to respond to stimuli), there is a reduced capacity to produce cyclic adenosine monophosphate (cAMP), and calcium ion channels become closed.

- The result is opioid intoxication: central nervous system and respiratory depression, lowered blood pressure, euphoria, miosis, nausea and vomiting, decreased peristalsis, and analgesia. In overdose, coma, respiratory arrest, pulmonary edema, profound hypotension, and hypoxic seizures can be seen
        - Long-term effects of opioid abuse include heart valve infections, infectious diseases (e.g. hepatitis A and C and HIV) that occur with IV use, arthritis, collapsed and sclerotic veins, malnutrition, and a depressed immune system ("Chemical Dependency")
    - Sedatives/Hypnotics
        - This is a large group of drugs that includes the most commonly abused barbiturates and benzodiazepines.
        - Barbiturates and benzodiazepines work by binding to specific barbiturate and benzodiazepine receptors.
        - This enhances the activity of the inhibitory neurotransmitter GABA, which then increases the frequency or duration of the opening of chloride channels and hyperpolarizes the cell.
        - The clinical effects of these drugs include central and respiratory system depression, ataxia, confusion, slurred speech, and impaired coordination. When taken in dangerous doses, coma and respiratory arrest are possible.
        - Long-term effects include tolerance, impaired memory and coordination, confusion, and disorientation ("Chemical Dependency")

Treatment

- Complex process; early prevention measures may be more successful
- Detoxification is the first step in treating chemical dependency, and it involves stopping the use of the drug and managing the signs and symptoms of withdrawal.
    - Alcohol withdrawal: Withdrawal signs and symptoms from alcohol can occur as soon as 4-6 hours after the last drink, but the onset may be delayed by 7-10 days.
        - The signs and symptoms can be mild (anxiety, irritability, depression, fatigue), moderate (diaphoresis, insomnia, elevated heart rate and blood pressure), or severe (severe confusion and hallucinations [delirium tremens], fever, convulsions).
        - Treatment consists of supportive care, fluid replacement when necessary, providing a safe environment, correcting electrolyte abnormalities, and administering a multivitamin and thiamine.
        - Benzodiazepines enhance the activity of GABA and are the first-line drug therapy; other medications that can be used are beta-blockers, α-blockers such as clonidine, anticonvulsants (e.g. carbamazapine), and neuroleptics.
        - Antipsychotics (e.g. haloperidol) can lower the seizure threshold and should be used with caution.

- Amphetamine withdrawal: There is no clear-cut evidence that explains the signs and symptoms of amphetamine withdrawal.
    - Symptoms of amphetamine withdrawal may include anxiety, nausea, palpitations, and irritability.
    - Currently, there are no approved methods for treating amphetamine withdrawal, but it is not generally considered to be dangerous and can be managed using benzodiazepines and symptomatic/supportive care.
- Benzodiazepine/barbiturate withdrawal: Although many cases of benzodiazepine withdrawal are relatively benign, withdrawal from these drugs can be severe, and fever, tachycardia, hypertension, and seizures are not unknown ("Chemical Dependency").
    - The classic approach to treating benzodiazepine withdrawal has been to use gradually tapering doses of benzodiazepines (either a fixed dose or a symptom-based dose), but there have been failures using this approach.
    - Tricyclic antidepressants, propranolol, progesterone, and buspirone have not proved effective, but the anticonvulsant carbamazepine may help.
- Cocaine withdrawal: The effects of cocaine withdrawal are thought to be due to a decreased release of dopamine and serotonin.
    - Cocaine withdrawal signs and symptoms include depression, fatigue, agitation, and general malaise; withdrawal from this drug is not considered to be medically dangerous.
    - It is generally managed with symptomatic and supportive care. There has been some experience in managing cocaine withdrawal using modafinil, a central nervous system stimulant that is currently used to treat narcolepsy.
    - Some clinicians have reported success in treating cocaine withdrawal using propranolol.
- Heroin withdrawal: Heroin withdrawal is uncomfortable (nausea, vomiting, diarrhea, anxiety, and palpitations), but not dangerous.
    - It is generally treated with symptomatic/supportive care, drugs such as the synthetic opioids methadone and buprenorphine, and the α-antagonist clonidine.
    - In recent years, there has been much attention focused on ultra-rapid opioid detoxification.
    - In this procedure, general anesthesia is used, and the opioid antagonist naltrexone is administered while the patient is unconscious. This approach is alluring; however, it is expensive, there are significant potential adverse effects, and there is no evidence that it is more effective than far less risky approaches (Harvard University, 2004).

Pharmacological Therapy

- Patients with heroin and alcohol dependency respond well to medication management.
- Medications to treat alcoholism (disulfiram, Naltrexone, Acamprosate, Carbamazepine, valproic acid, and topirimate) prevent the metabolism of alcohol.

- Treatment for opioid dependence has traditionally relied on a synthetic opioid, methadone.
- Methadone has a much longer duration of action than other opioids, thus eliminating the rapid shifts between "highs" and the absence of an opioid.
- Buprenorphine is a *mu* opiate receptor partial agonist, and clinical studies have shown that it can reduce the abuse of illicit opiates and reduce cravings.
- There are no approved pharmacological treatments for cocaine dependency ("Chemical Dependency").

Psychological Therapy

- No consensus as to what is the "best" psychological approach for treating chemical dependency
- Behavioral therapy
- Cognitive behavioral therapy - grounded in social learning theories and operant conditioning
- Contingency management - in this technique, patients receive rewards for specific behavioral goals; there is a lot of very good empirical support for its effectiveness
- Motivational interviewing - a focused, goal-directed technique that helps patients explore and resolve ambivalence and helps patients toward an acceptable goal ("Chemical Dependency")

Nursing Considerations

- Hope and optimism: Given the seemingly self-inflicted nature of chemical dependency and the high relapse rate, it can be a challenge to remain hopeful and optimistic, but these attitudes are essential.
- A non-judgmental attitude: It is very easy to form judgments about patients with chemical dependency and to view them as weak or lacking in morals and/or self-control.
- A low need to control the patient
- The ability to engage the patient, but still remain detached
- Patience and tolerance: Chemical dependency is a chronic disease, and relapses are very common.
- Flexibility
- Recognize that people with chemical dependency often have co-occurring psychiatric disorders that must be treated ("Chemical Dependency").

List of Nursing Interventions by Domain

Domain 1: Basic Physiological
- Activity/Exercise Management
- Elimination Management
- Immobility Management
- Nutritional Support

- Physical Comfort Promotion
- Self-care Facilitation

Domain 2: Complex Physiological
- Electrolyte & Acid-base Management
- Drug Management
- Neurological Management
- Perioperative Care
- Respiratory Management
- Skin/Wound Management
- Thermoregulation
- Tissue Perfusion Management

Domain 3: Behavioral
- Behavior Therapy
- Cognitive Therapy
- Communication Enhancement
- Coping Assistance
- Patient Education
- Psychological Comfort Promotion

Domain 4: Family
- Lifespan Care

Domain 5: Safety
- Crisis Management
- Risk Management

Domain 6: Health System
- Health System Mediation
- Health System Management

Test Your Knowledge

1. Early lab results that are definitive of herpes simplex encephalitis include:
    a. Viral DNA found in the CSF
    b. CT scan of the brain
    c. Characteristic temporal sharp waves seen on the EEG
    d. A fourfold increase in serum antibody titer

2. What nutritional advice is best for a patient who will be discharged with Coumadin to prevent recurrence of embolic stroke?
    a. Green leafy vegetables are okay to eat regularly and in moderation.
    b. Iron supplements are advised to counteract the anemia associated with silent microscopic GI bleeding.
    c. Take vitamin K supplement because Coumadin inhibits vitamin K.
    d. Do not drink more than two glasses of wine or one mixed drink per week.

3. Your patient is about to undergo a lumbar puncture at bedside. What is the most important part of your nursing preparation?
    a. Keeping the patient NPO for the next three hours.
    b. Check coagulation panel and platelet count.
    c. Educate patient and family about procedure and possible complications during procedure.
    d. Have patient use bathroom to empty bladder prior to procedure.

4. Antibiotic therapy is an important aspect of care for a patient with bacterial meningitis. Which statement below is reflective of antibiotic therapy?
    a. Antibiotics should be given prior to giving any steroids.
    b. Do not administer antibiotics until specific disease-causing organism has been identified.
    c. Initial antibiotics are based on the most likely causative agent and should be reassessed as soon as CSF lab results return.
    d. Bacteriostatic and bactericidal types of antibiotics are equally acceptable.

5. A patient is being discharged from the hospital after an early diagnosis and treatment of Lyme disease. What is an important element of education for this patient?
    a. Inform the patient about the long-term effects of disease including joint damage.
    b. Educate the patient regarding the use of isolation until all antibiotics are complete.
    c. Stress the importance of finishing all antibiotics.
    d. Reassure the patient that he/she has conferred immunity to B. burgdorferi, the causative agent of Lyme disease.

6. When caring for a patient with viral meningitis, which of the following is not an important nursing intervention?
   a. Keep patient in isolation until he/she is afebrile without antipyretics for at least 24 hours.
   b. Keep room cool to avoid hyperthermia, apply cool clothes to head, and take antipyretics as necessary.
   c. Assess neurological status frequently to detect ALOC or focal abnormalities.
   d. Implement steps to prevent increased ICP. Maintain head and neck in alignment and start bowel program to prevent stimulating the Valsalva response.

7. You are a nurse working in the emergency department when a college student is brought in with fever, severe headache, and weird/strange behavior. The symptoms have been present the last few hours. The conjunctiva and skin show petechiae. What is the most URGENT supportive measure needed to prepare the patient for a lumbar puncture?
   a. Administer antipyretics.
   b. Prepare for intubation.
   c. Provide adequate IV access.
   d. Educate patient and roommate about meningitis vaccination.

8. A patient with multiple sclerosis is about to start an exercise class. The most effective way to cool core body temperature during exercise is:
   a. Wear a cooling vest.
   b. Dress in light clothes.
   c. Drink cool liquids.
   d. Prior to exercise, take antipyretics.

9. Your patient Helen has relapsing multiple sclerosis. She has told you that she would like to stop taking interferon beta-1b. She stated that there have been no improvements since starting the medications several years ago. The most appropriate response is:
   a. Suggest changing to interferon beta-1a or glatiramer acetate.
   b. Since depression is a known side effect of interferon therapy and a symptom of multiple sclerosis, evaluate her for depression.
   c. Explain to her that the goals of therapy are to delay disability development and to decrease the frequency and severity of exacerbations; provide regular phone calls with follow-up to support her in continuing the treatment.
   d. Assist with the management of flu-like symptoms by pretreating with NSAIDS or Tylenol.

10. Your patient is diagnosed with myasthenia gravis. What is the best dietary advice to give him/her?
    a. Do not eat if fatigued.
    b. Take anti-cholinergic medication before every meal.
    c. Consume a liquid diet on days when the muscles of mastication feel weak.
    d. Eat small meals that are mechanically soft.

11. Which is the most accurate statement concerning antibiotic therapy for bacterial meningitis?
    a. Treatment should not commence until the causative organism has been identified.
    b. Bactericidal and bacteriostatic antibiotics are equally acceptable.
    c. Initial drug selection is based on the most likely organisms and should be reassessed within hours when CSF laboratory results return.
    d. Antibiotic therapy should be initiated before administering any dexamethasone.

12. Which of the following is NOT an important nursing intervention in the care of a patient with viral meningitis?
    a. Serial neurological examinations to detect focal abnormalities or altered consciousness.
    b. Taking steps to prevent increased intracranial pressure such as maintaining the neck in neutral position and instituting a good bowel program to prevent the need for Valsalva.
    c. Avoiding hyperthermia by keeping the room cool, applying moist cloths to the head, and administering antipyretic drugs as necessary.
    d. Maintaining isolation until the patient has been afebrile without antipyretic drugs for at least 24 hours.

13. The MOST important part of nursing preparation for a patient about to undergo diagnostic lumbar puncture is:
    a. Check platelet count and coagulation studies.
    b. Have the patient empty his/her bladder and move his/her bowel if possible.
    c. Maintain the patient NPO for six hours or more.
    d. Educate the patient about the purpose, method, and possible complications of the procedure.

14. The MOST important element of assessment of the patient hospitalized for worsening myasthenia is:
    a. Comprehensive assessment of respiratory function.
    b. Evaluation of voice quality and volume.
    c. Evaluation of extraocular muscle function.
    d. Avoidance of neuromuscular-blocking drugs.

15. Pro-active decision making about life supports such as gastrostomy for feeding or tracheostomy for ventilation is essential for patients with amyotrophic lateral sclerosis (ALS) because:
    a. Death from ALS most commonly occurs because of aspiration or respiratory failure.
    b. When terminal, an ALS patient may be unable to communicate.
    c. ALS is a progressive disease, and 50% of the patients die within three years of diagnosis.
    d. For ALS patients, feeding tubes and artificial ventilation are not temporary life-saving measures that can be instituted and then withdrawn when a crisis resolves.

16. Which of the following represents the approximate number of ischemic strokes that occur each year in the U.S.?
    a. 700,000
    b. 400,000
    c. 50,000
    d. 45,000

17. Which of the following is the main cause of an ischemic stroke?
    a. An interruption in the blood supply to the brain
    b. A burst blood vessel in the brain
    c. A tumor mass in the brain
    d. A ruptured aneurysm

18. Cardiac sources of embolic stroke include which of the following?
    a. Patent foramen ovale and cocaine use
    b. Carotid dissection and cocaine use
    c. Cerebral aneurysm and atrial fibrillation
    d. Atrial fibrillation and patent foramen ovale

19. Conditions that can mimic an ischemic stroke include which of the following?
    a. Hypoglycemia and unrecognized seizures
    b. Cardiac arrest and hypoglycemia
    c. Unrecognized seizures and fatigue
    d. Hemiplegia and heart attack

20. The nurse in the emergency department should plan for which initial tests for all patients suspected of acute ischemic stroke?
    a. Urgent EEG
    b. Lipid profile
    c. Lumbar puncture
    d. Non-contrast brain CT scan

21. Which of the following would exclude a patient with acute ischemic stroke from receiving IV tPA?
    a. NIHSS = 16
    b. BP = 185/100 mm Hg
    c. Blood glucose = 40 mg/dl
    d. INR = 1.2

22. Which of the following treatments can extend the three-hour window of acute-therapy to 12 hours?
    a. Anticoagulation
    b. IA thrombolysis
    c. IVIG therapy
    d. IV steroids

23. A 68-year-old male patient is admitted to the acute stroke unit for IV tPA with a BP of 195/110 mm HG and blood glucose of 120mg/dl. Which of the following should the nurse do first?
    a. Prepare to administer 10-20 mg IV Labetalol.
    b. Do a full neurological examination.
    c. Prepare to administer nitropaste two inches.
    d. Re-check the blood glucose level.

24. Prevention of acute complications for patients with ischemic stroke includes which of the following?
    a. Hypothermia and monitoring for cardiac dysrhythmias
    b. Intubation and hypertension management
    c. Monitoring for fever and cardiac dysrhythmias
    d. Albumin and medications to increase BP

25. The nurse is assessing risk factors for a 55-year-old woman who has had an ischemic stroke and has a waist circumference of 45 inches. Which of the following is the most accurate secondary stroke prevention guideline for this patient?
    a. There are no waist circumference guidelines.
    b. A waist circumference of < 40 inches is advised.
    c. Physical exercise of 45 minutes per day is advised.
    d. A waist circumference of < 35 inches is advised.

26. What is the type of mechanism of injury related to TBIs that involves damage to the blood-brain barrier and tiny cerebral blood vessels, which are caused by the blood surge moving quickly through large blood vessels to the brain from the torso?
    a. Penetrating
    b. Blast
    c. Blunt
    d. Accelerated

27. Which statement best describes the clinical sequelae related to secondary injury sustained with a traumatic brain injury?
    a. Many of those with TBI who survive emergency department arrival will still die within a matter of days or weeks as a result of secondary brain injury.
    b. Defined as any complicating injury that occurs as a result of further physiological events at some point later in the clinical course.
    c. Can result from a single neurological event, a series of events, or multisystem complications.
    d. All of the above

28. Upon presentation to the emergency department, EMS reports to the primary nurse the patient's initial GCS score of 3, that the patient was unable to maintain airway, and that he showed signs of flexor posturing. Given the clinical presentation, the nurse concludes the patient has sustained which type of head injury?
    a. Minor head injury
    b. Moderate head injury
    c. Severe head injury
    d. None of the above

29. A patient is admitted with a sub-acute subdural hematoma. The nurse realizes this patient will most likely be treated with:
    a. Emergency craniotomy
    b. Elective draining of the hematoma
    c. Burr holes to remove the hematoma
    d. Removal of the affected cranial lobe

30. While undergoing morning care, a patient begins to have a seizure. Which of the following should the nurse do?
    a. Protect the patient's head and other body parts from injury
    b. Insert a tongue blade into the patient's mouth
    c. Call for someone to bring an oral airway to insert into the patient's mouth
    d. Hold the patient's arms

31. During the hourly neurological assessment, a patient is demonstrating signs of the Cushing response. These signs include:
    a. Tachycardia
    b. Hyperventilation
    c. Hypoventilation
    d. Hypotension

32. A patient's oxygen level is dropping. The nurse realizes that because of cerebral auto-regulation, the following will occur:
    a. Cerebral blood vessels will dilate
    b. Cerebral blood vessels will constrict
    c. Blood will be shunted from the cerebral cortex
    d. Blood flow to the cerebral cortex will slow

33. The nurse is providing discharge instructions to a patient with a mild brain injury. Which of the following should be included in these instructions?
    a. The headache will go away in a few days.
    b. Return to normal activities and work.
    c. Avoid participating in activities that caused the injury because of a cumulative effect.
    d. Dizziness will disappear in a few days.

34. A patient with a traumatic brain injury is in need of fluid replacement therapy to maintain a systolic blood pressure of at least 90 mm Hg. The nurse realizes that the best fluid replacement for this patient would be:
    a. 0.9% normal saline (NS)
    b. D5W
    c. D5 and 0.45% normal saline (NS)
    d. 0.45% normal saline (NS)

35. The nurse is providing care to a patient with a traumatic brain injury. Nutritional intervention for this patient would include:
    a. Full parenteral nutrition
    b. Enteral feedings initiated 24 hours after injury
    c. Enteral feedings initiated 72 hours after injury
    d. Enteral feedings stopped by the seventh day after injury

36. Coma stimulation is being implemented for a patient who sustained a traumatic brain injury. Which of the following should be included in this plan for stimulation?
    a. Provide stimulation before a sleep/rest period.
    b. Stop the family from bringing in personal items of the patient.
    c. Increase the volume level of speaking and stimulation in the patient's room.
    d. Ensure that only one person at a time is speaking during the period of stimulation.

37. Which instruction is most appropriate to prevent triggering the pain in patients with trigeminal neuralgia?
    a. Eat iced foods
    b. Avoid oral hygiene
    c. Apply warm compresses
    d. Chew on the unaffected side

38. Broca's (motor) aphasia refers to:
    a. Inability to understand spoken language
    b. Fluent, nonsensical speech
    c. Fluent, sensical speech
    d. Inability to express yourself

39. A technique used to assess language dominance and memory function before ablative surgery for epilepsy is:
    a. Magnetoencephalogram
    b. Intracarotid Amobarbital Procedure (Wada Test)
    c. Visual-evoked potential
    d. Somatosensory evoked potential

40. Glasgow Coma Scale (GCS) is a measure of :
    a. Level of consciousness (LOC)
    b. Memory
    c. Intracranial pressure (ICP)
    d. Fluid volume

41. Therapeutic intervention for increased intra cranial pressure (ICP) includes all the following except:
    a. Administer mannitol, an osmotic diuretic
    b. Administer hypertonic saline
    c. Administer corticosteroids
    d. Hyperventilation

42. Fever, headache, and nuchal rigidity are classic symptoms seen in:
    a. Parkinson's disease
    b. Alzheimer's disease
    c. Brain abscess
    d. Meningitis

43. A condition characterized by the occurrence of small patches of demyelination of the white matter of the optic nerve, brain, and spinal cord is:
    a. Amyotrophic lateral sclerosis (ALS)
    b. Multiple sclerosis (MS)
    c. Lou Gehrig's disease
    d. Parkinson's disease
    e. Alzheimer's disease

44. The part of the neuron that receives messages from other cells is called:
    a. Axon
    b. Soma
    c. Schwann cell
    d. Dendrites

45. Which of the following is a specific investigation to detect seizures?
    a. CT scan
    b. MRI scan
    c. EEG
    d. BEAP

46. The most common inhibitory neurotransmitter in the human brain is:
    a. Acetylcholine
    b. Serotonin
    c. GABA
    d. Dopamine

47. Which of the following medications may retard the progress of Alzheimer's disease deterioration?
    a. Donepezil
    b. L-dopa
    c. Prednisone
    d. Vitamin B12

48. Parkinson's disease is caused by the degeneration of neurons in an area of the brain called the:
    a. Substantia nigra
    b. Basal ganglia
    c. Cerebellum
    d. Corpus callosum

49. A condition causing the affected person to be unable to understand or comprehend the language (poor comprehension) with intact repetition (fluent output) is:
    a. Broca's aphasia
    b. Global aphasia
    c. Wernicke's aphasia
    d. Conduction aphasia

50. Symptoms of Parkinson's disease include all of the following except:
    a. Tremors of the hands, arms, legs, jaw, and face
    b. Stiff limbs
    c. Bradykinesia and impaired balance
    d. Impaired cognition

51. Treatment for epilepsy to eliminate or sharply reduce the frequency of seizures may involve all of the following except:
    a. Cognitive-behavioral therapy
    b. Narrow-spectrum and broad-spectrum antiepileptic drugs
    c. Vagus-nerve stimulation
    d. Surgery

52. All of the following may be associated with Guillain-Barré Syndrome except:
    a. Weakening or tingling sensation in the legs
    b. Weakness in the arms and upper body
    c. Nearly complete paralysis
    d. First symptom is altered mental status

53. Gradually increasing pain and weakness and numbness in the hand or wrist that radiates up the arm suggest:
    a. Amyotrophic lateral sclerosis
    b. Carpal tunnel syndrome
    c. Bloch-Sulzberger syndrome
    d. Dystonia

54. Difficulty speaking and understanding speech is termed:
    a. Apnea
    b. Ataxia
    c. Aphasia
    d. Dyslexia

55. A male client has an impairment of cranial nerve II. Specific to this impairment, the nurse would plan to do which of the following to ensure client safety?
    a. Speak loudly to the client
    b. Test the temperature of the shower water
    c. Check the temperature of the food on the delivery tray
    d. Provide a clear path without obstacles for ambulation

56. The most common cause of subarachnoid hemorrhage is:
    a. Aneurysms
    b. Coagulopathies
    c. Trauma from falls
    d. Ischemia

57. Which of the following statements best describes transient ischemic attacks (TIAs)?
    a. Damage and symptoms resolve.
    b. Damage and symptoms are permanent.
    c. Damage is permanent, but symptoms resolve.
    d. Damage is permanent, but there are no symptoms.

58. The best indicator of changes in neurological function in an alert patient is:
    a. Changes in behavior
    b. Disorientation
    c. Unresponsiveness
    d. Pupil changes

59. Nursing intervention for the neuro patient should include:
    a. Not clustering activities
    b. Performing frequent neuro checks
    c. Administering diuretics
    d. Positioning in the prone position

60. Brief loss of consciousness followed by a lucid period and a secondary loss of consciousness is characteristic of which traumatic brain injury?
    a. Subdural hematoma
    b. Subarachnoid hemorrhage
    c. Epidural hemorrhage
    d. Concussion

61. In a patient with increased intracranial pressure, cerebral perfusion pressure should be maintained at:
    a. 40 mm Hg
    b. 50 mm Hg
    c. 60 mm Hg
    d. 70 mm Hg

62. The most sensitive indicator of changes in intracranial pressure in unresponsive patients is:
    a. Change in systolic blood pressure
    b. Change in pupil response
    c. Blood glucose levels
    d. Response of the cranial nerves

63. You are helping a patient with a spinal cord injury (SCI) to establish a bladder-retraining program. Which of the following strategies will not stimulate the patient to void?
    a. Stroke the patient's inner thigh.
    b. Pull on the patient's pubic hair.
    c. Initiate intermittent straight catheterization.
    d. Pour warm water over the perineum.
    e. Tap the bladder to stimulate detrusor muscle.

64. A patient with a spinal cord injury (SCI) complains about a severe throbbing headache that suddenly started a short time ago. Assessment of the patient reveals increased blood pressure (168/94) and decreased heart rate (48/minute), diaphoresis, and flushing of the face and neck. Which action should you take first?
    a. Administer the ordered acetaminophen (Tylenol).
    b. Check the Foley tubing for kinks or obstruction.
    c. Adjust the temperature in the patient's room.
    d. Notify the physician about the change in status.

65. The patient with multiple sclerosis tells the nursing assistant that after physical therapy she is too tired to take a bath. What is your priority nursing diagnosis at this time?
    a. Fatigue related to disease state
    b. Activity intolerance due to generalized weakness
    c. Impaired physical mobility related to neuromuscular impairment
    d. Self-care deficit related to fatigue and neuromuscular weakness

66. You are caring for a patient with an acute hemorrhagic stroke. The patient's husband has been reading a lot about strokes and asks why his wife did not receive alteplase. What is your best response?
    a. "Your wife was not admitted within the time frame that alteplase is usually given."
    b. "This drug is used primarily for patients who experience an acute heart attack."
    c. "Alteplase dissolves clots and may cause more bleeding into your wife's brain."
    d. "Your wife had gallbladder surgery just six months ago, which prevents the use of alteplase."

67. A stroke patient needs to be fed. Which instruction should you give to the nursing assistant who will feed the patient?
    a. Before you feed the patient, position her sitting up in bed.
    b. Check the patient's gag and swallowing reflexes.
    c. Feed the patient quickly because there are three more patients waiting.
    d. Suction the patient's secretions between bites of food.

68. You have just admitted a patient with bacterial meningitis to the medical-surgical unit. The patient complains of a severe headache with photophobia and has an oral temperature of 102.6° F. Which collaborative intervention must be completed first?
    a. Administer codeine 15 mg orally for the patient's headache.
    b. Infuse ceftriaxone (Rocephin) 2,000 mg IV to treat the infection.
    c. Give acetaminophen (Tylenol) 650 mg orally to reduce the fever.
    d. Give furosemide (Lasix) 40 mg IV to decrease intracranial pressure.

69. A patient who has recently started phenytoin (Dilantin) to control simple complex seizures is seen in the outpatient clinic. Which information obtained during his chart review and assessment will be of greatest concern?
    a. The gums appear enlarged and inflamed.
    b. The white blood cell count is 2300/mm3.
    c. Patient occasionally forgets to take phenytoin until after lunch.
    d. Patient wants to renew his driver's license in the next month.

70. You are caring for a patient with a recurrent glioblastoma who is receiving dexamethasone (Decadron) 4 mg IV every six hours to relieve symptoms of right arm weakness and headache. Which assessment information concerns you the most?
    a. The patient does not recognize family members.
    b. The blood glucose level is 234 mg/dL.
    c. The patient complains of a continued headache.
    d. The daily weight has increased 1 kg.

71. A 70-year-old alcoholic patient with acute lethargy, confusion, and incontinence is admitted to the hospital emergency department. His wife tells you that he fell down the stairs about a month ago, but "he didn't have a scratch afterward." She feels that he has become gradually less active and sleepier over the last 10 days or so. Which of the following collaborative interventions should you implement first?
    a. Place on the hospital alcohol withdrawal protocol
    b. Transfer to radiology for a CT scan
    c. Insert a retention catheter to straight drainage
    d. Give phenytoin (Dilantin) 100 mg PO

72. You are mentoring a student nurse in the intensive care unit (ICU) while caring for a patient with meningococcal meningitis. Which action by the student requires that you intervene immediately?
    a. The student enters the room without putting on a mask and gown.
    b. The student instructs the family that visits are restricted to 10 minutes.
    c. The student gives the patient a warm blanket when he says he feels cold.
    d. The student checks the patient's pupil response to light every 30 minutes.

73. You are creating a teaching plan for a patient with newly diagnosed migraine headaches. Which of the following should be included in the teaching plan?
    a. Avoid foods that contain tyramine such as alcohol and aged cheese.
    b. Avoid drugs such as Tagamet, nitroglycerin, and Nifedipine.
    c. Abortive therapy is aimed at eliminating the pain during the aura.
    d. A potential side effect of medications is rebound headache.
    e. Complementary therapies such as relaxation may be helpful.
    f. All of the above

74. A client is admitted to an emergency department. A nurse in the emergency department documents that the client is "postictal upon transfer" as evidenced by which observation?
    a. Yellowing of the skin
    b. Recently experienced a seizure and is in a drowsy or confused state
    c. Severe itching of the eyes
    d. Abnormal sensations including tingling of the skin

75. A client has a hearing loss from a suspected acoustic neuroma. Which diagnostic test should a nurse plan to prepare the client to confirm the presence of a tumor?
    a. Tympanometry
    b. Arteriogram of the cranial vessels
    c. Magnetic resonance imaging (MRI)
    d. Auditory canal biopsy

76. A _____ injury is one in which the scalp and skull remain intact, but the underlying tissue is damaged.
    a. Open
    b. Linear
    c. Depressed
    d. Closed

77. An excessive accumulation of cerebrospinal fluid (CSF) is known as:
    a. Cushing's Triad
    b. Ipsilateral
    c. Subdural hematoma
    d. Hydrocephalus

78. A chronic disturbance of the nervous system characterized by recurrent seizures that are the result of abnormal electrical activity of the brain is known as:
    a. Parkinson's disease
    b. Lou Gehrig's disease
    c. Epilepsy
    d. Guillain- Barré

79. When the brain tissue is bruised, blood from the broken vessels accumulates and edema develops, causing increased intracranial pressure (ICP). This injury is known as:
    a. Closed
    b. Ipsilateral
    c. Subluxation
    d. Contusion

80. When admitting a patient who has a tumor of the right frontal lobe, the nurse would expect to find:
    a. Short-term memory
    b. Judgment changes
    c. Swallowing changes
    d. Speech difficulties

81. While admitting a patient with a basal skull fracture, the nurse sees clear drainage from the patient's nose. Which of these admission orders should the nurse question?
    a. Insert nasogastric tube
    b. Check nasal drainage for glucose
    c. Mannitol IV
    d. Neuro checks every hour for 24 hours

82. A patient with a neck fracture at the C5 level is admitted to the intensive care unit. During initial assessment of the patient, the nurse recognizes the presence of neurogenic shock on finding:
    a. The patient takes warfarin (Coumadin) daily.
    b. The patient has hypotension, bradycardia, and warm extremities.
    c. The patient exhibits spasticity and hyperactive reflexes.
    d. The patient has elevated blood pressure and respirations.

83. A patient with a head injury opens his eyes to verbal stimulation, curses when stimulated, and does not respond to a verbal command to move, but attempts to remove the painful stimulus. The nurse records the patient's Glasgow Coma Scale score as:
    a. 18
    b. 11
    c. 3
    d. 8

84. The nurse recognizes the presence of Cushing's triad in the patient with:
    a. Increased pulse, irregular respiration, increased blood pressure
    b. Decreased pulse, irregular respiration, increased pulse pressure
    c. Increased pulse, decreased respiration, increased pulse pressure
    d. Decreased pulse, increased respiration, decreased systolic blood pressure

85. A patient has intracranial pressure (ICP) monitoring with an intraventricular catheter. A priority nursing intervention for the patient is:
    a. Aseptic technique to prevent infection
    b. Constant monitoring of ICP waveforms
    c. Removal of CSF to maintain normal ICP
    d. Sampling CSF to determine abnormalities

86. Metabolic and nutritional needs of the patient with increased ICP are best met with:
    a. Enteral feedings low in sodium
    b. The simple glucose available in D5W IV solutions
    c. A fluid restriction that promotes moderate dehydration
    d. Balanced, essential nutrition in a form the patient can tolerate

87. Cranial nerve three (CN III) originating in the midbrain is assessed by the nurse for an early indication of pressure on the brainstem by:
    a. Assessing for nystagmus
    b. Testing the corneal reflex
    c. Testing pupillary reaction to light
    d. Testing for oculocephalic (doll's eye) reflex

88. A patient has a nursing diagnosis of risk for ineffective cerebral tissue perfusion related to cerebral edema. An appropriate nursing intervention for the patient is:
    a. Avoid positioning the patient with neck and hip flexion
    b. Maintain hyperventilation to a PaCO2 of 15-20 mm Hg
    c. Cluster nursing activities to provide periods of uninterrupted rest
    d. Routine suctioning to prevent accumulation of respiratory secretions

89. While the nurse performs range of motion (ROM) exercises on an unconscious patient with increased intracranial pressure (ICP), the patient experiences severe decerebrate posturing reflexes. The nurse should:
    a. Use restraints to protect the patient from injury
    b. Administer CNS depressants to lightly sedate the patient
    c. Perform the exercises less frequently because posturing can increase ICP
    d. Continue the exercises because they are necessary to maintain musculoskeletal function

90. The nurse suspects the presence of an arterial epidural hematoma in the patient who experiences:
    a. Failure to regain consciousness following a head injury
    b. A rapid deterioration of neurologic function within 24 to 48 hours following a head injury
    c. Non-specific, non-localizing progression of alteration in level of consciousness (LOC) occurring over weeks or months
    d. Unconsciousness at the time of a head injury with a brief period of consciousness followed by a decrease in level of consciousness (LOC)

91. Skull radiographs and a CT scan provide evidence of a depressed parietal fracture with a subdural hematoma in a patient admitted to the emergency department following an automobile accident. In planning care for the patient, the nurse anticipates that:
    a. The patient will receive life-support measures until the condition stabilizes
    b. Immediate burr holes will be made to rapidly decompress the intracranial activity
    c. The patient will be treated conservatively with close monitoring for changes in neurologic condition
    d. The patient will be taken to surgery for a craniotomy for evacuation of blood and decompression of the cranium

92. When a patient is admitted to the emergency department following a head injury, the nurse's first priority in management of the patient once a patent airway is confirmed is:
    a. Maintaining cervical spine precautions
    b. Determining the presence of increased ICP
    c. Monitoring for changes in neurologic status
    d. Establishing IV access with a large-bore catheter

93. Assisting the family to understand what is happening to the patient is an especially important role of the nurse when the patient has a tumor of the:
    a. Ventricles
    b. Frontal lobe
    c. Parietal lobe
    d. Occipital lobe

94. Classic symptoms of bacterial meningitis include:
    a. Papilledema and psychomotor seizures
    b. High fever, nuchal rigidity, and severe headache
    c. Behavioral changes with memory loss and lethargy
    d. Positive Kernig's and Brudzinski's signs and hemiparesis

95. The nurse plans care for a patient with increased ICP with the knowledge that the best way to position the patient is to:
    a. Keep the head of the bed flat
    b. Elevate the head of the bed to 30°
    c. Maintain patient on the left side with the head supported on a pillow
    d. Use a continuous rotation bed to continuously change patient position

96. A nurse on a clinical unit is assigned to four patients. Which patient should she assess first?
    a. Patient with a skull fracture whose nose is bleeding
    b. Elderly patient with a stroke who is confused and whose daughter is present
    c. Patient with meningitis who is suddenly agitated and reporting a headache of 10 on a 0 to 10 scale
    d. Patient who had a craniotomy for a brain tumor who is now three days post-operative and has had continued emesis

97. Which domain of nursing interventions includes crisis management and risk management?
    a. Domain 1: Basic Physiological
    b. Domain 3: Behavioral
    c. Domain 4: Family
    d. Domain 5: Safety

98. The nurse is teaching a female client with multiple sclerosis. When teaching the client how to reduce fatigue, the nurse should tell the client to:
    a. Take a hot bath
    b. Rest in an air-conditioned room
    c. Increase the dose of muscle relaxants
    d. Avoid naps during the day

99. A female client with Guillain-Barré syndrome has paralysis affecting the respiratory muscles and requires mechanical ventilation. When the client asks the nurse about the paralysis, how should the nurse respond?
   a. "You may have difficulty believing this, but the paralysis caused by this disease is temporary."
   b. "You'll have to accept the fact that you're permanently paralyzed. However, you won't have any sensory loss."
   c. "It must be hard to accept the permanency of your paralysis."
   d. "You'll first regain use of your legs and then your arms."

100. A nurse is working on a surgical floor. The nurse must logroll a male client following a:
   a. Laminectomy
   b. Thoracotomy
   c. Hemorrhoidectomy
   d. Cystectomy

101. A female client with a suspected brain tumor is scheduled for a CT scan. What should the nurse do when preparing the client for this test?
   a. Immobilize the neck before the client is moved onto a stretcher
   b. Determine whether the client is allergic to iodine, contrast dyes, or shellfish
   c. Place a cap over the client's head
   d. Administer a sedative as ordered

102. During a routine physical examination to assess a male client's deep tendon reflexes, the nurse should make sure to:
   a. Use the pointed end of the reflex hammer when striking the Achilles tendon
   b. Support the joint where the tendon is being tested
   c. Tap the tendon slowly and softly
   d. Hold the reflex hammer tightly

103. A female client is admitted in a disoriented and restless state after sustaining a concussion during a car accident. Which nursing diagnosis takes the highest priority in this client's plan of care?
   a. Disturbed sensory perception (visual)
   b. Self-care deficient: dressing/grooming
   c. Impaired verbal communication
   d. Risk for injury

104. A female client with amyotrophic lateral sclerosis (ALS) tells the nurse, "Sometimes I feel so frustrated. I can't do anything without help!" This comment best supports which nursing diagnosis?
    a. Anxiety
    b. Powerlessness
    c. Ineffective denial
    d. Risk for disuse syndrome

105. A female client admitted to the hospital with a neurological problem asks the nurse whether magnetic resonance imaging may be done. The nurse interprets that the client may be ineligible for this diagnostic procedure based on the client's history of:
    a. Hypertension
    b. Heart failure
    c. Prosthetic valve replacement
    d. Chronic obstructive pulmonary disorder

106. A male client is having a lumbar puncture performed. The nurse would plan to place the client in which position?
    a. Side-lying with a pillow under the hip
    b. Prone with a pillow under the abdomen
    c. Prone in slight-Trendelenburg's position
    d. Side-lying with legs pulled up and head bent down onto chest

107. The nurse is positioning a female client with increased intracranial pressure. Which of the following positions would the nurse avoid?
    a. Head midline
    b. Head turned to side
    c. Neck in neutral position
    d. Head of bed elevated to 30 to 45°

108. A male client with a spinal cord injury is prone to experiencing automatic dysreflexia. Which of the following measures would the nurse avoid to minimize the risk of recurrence?
    a. Strict adherence to a bowel-retraining program
    b. Keeping the linen under the client wrinkle-free
    c. Preventing unnecessary pressure on the lower limbs
    d. Limiting bladder catheterization to once every 12 hours

109. The nurse is assigned to care for a female client with complete right-sided hemiparesis. The nurse plans care knowing that in this condition:
    a. The client has complete bilateral paralysis of the arms and legs
    b. The client has weakness on the right side of the body including the face and tongue
    c. The client has lost the ability to move the left arm, but is able to walk independently
    d. The client has lost the ability to move the right arm, but is able to walk independently

110. A client with a brain attack (stroke) has residual dysphagia. When a diet order is initiated, the nurse avoids doing which of the following?
    a. Giving the client thin liquids
    b. Thickening liquids to the consistency of oatmeal
    c. Placing food on the unaffected side of the mouth
    d. Allowing plenty of time for chewing and swallowing

111. The nurse is assessing the adaptation of the female client to changes in functional status after a brain attack (stroke). The nurse assesses that the client is adapting most successfully if the client:
    a. Gets angry with family if they interrupt a task
    b. Experiences bouts of depression and irritability
    c. Has difficulty using modified feeding utensils
    d. Consistently uses adaptive equipment when dressing herself

112. Nurse Kristine is trying to communicate with a client with a brain attack (stroke) and aphasia. Which of the following actions by the nurse would be least helpful to the client?
    a. Speaking to the client at a slower rate
    b. Allowing plenty of time for the client to respond
    c. Completing the sentences that the client cannot finish
    d. Looking directly at the client during attempts at speech

113. A female client has experienced an episode of myasthenic crisis. The nurse would assess whether the client has which of the following precipitating factors?
    a. Getting too little exercise
    b. Taking excess medication
    c. Omitting doses of medication
    d. Increasing intake of fatty foods

114. A male client with Bell's palsy asks the nurse what has caused this problem. The nurse's response is based on an understanding that the cause is:
    a. Unknown, but possibly includes ischemia, viral infection, or an autoimmune problem
    b. Unknown, but possibly includes long-term tissue malnutrition and cellular hypoxia
    c. Primarily genetic in origin and triggered by exposure to meningitis
    d. Primarily genetic in origin and triggered by exposure to neurotoxins

115. A patient comes to the emergency department immediately after experiencing numbness of the face and an inability to speak, but while the patient awaits examination, the symptoms disappear and the patient requests a discharge. The nurse stresses that it is important for the patient to be evaluated primarily because:
    a. The patient has probably experienced an asymptomatic lacunar stroke
    b. The symptoms are likely to return and progress to worsening neurologic deficit in the next 24 hours
    c. Neurologic deficits that are transient occur most often as a result of small hemorrhages that clot off
    d. The patient has probably experienced a transient ischemic attack (TIA), which is a sign of progressive cerebral vascular disease

116. A carotid endarterectomy is being considered as a treatment for a patient who has had several TIAs. The nurse explains to the patient that this surgery:
    a. Is used to restore blood to the brain following an obstruction of a cerebral artery
    b. Involves intracranial surgery to join a superficial extracranial artery to an intracranial artery
    c. Involves removing an atherosclerotic plaque in the carotid artery to prevent an impending stroke
    d. Is used to open a stenosis in a carotid artery with a balloon and stent to restore cerebral circulation

117. The priority intervention in the emergency department for a patient with a stroke is:
    a. Intravenous fluid replacement
    b. Administration of osmotic diuretics to reduce cerebral edema
    c. Initiation of hypothermia to decrease the oxygen needs of the brain
    d. Maintenance of respiratory function with a patent airway and oxygen administration

118. The incidence of ischemic stroke in patients with TIAs and other risk factors is reduced with administration of:
    a. Furosemide (Lasix)
    b. Lovastatin (Mevacor)
    c. Daily low-dose aspirin
    d. Nimodipine (Nimotop)

119. A diagnosis of a ruptured cerebral aneurysm has been made in a patient with manifestations of a stroke. The nurse anticipates that possible treatment options for the patient will include:
    a. Hyperventilation therapy
    b. Surgical clipping of the aneurysm
    c. Administration of hyperosmotic agents
    d. Administration of thrombolytic therapy

120. Which of the following is the best treatment for acute ischemic stroke?
    a. Heparin
    b. LMWH
    c. Alteplase
    d. Eptifibatide
    e. Warfarin

Test Your Knowledge—Answers

1. a.
   One of the early lab results that is definitive of herpes simplex encephalitis is viral DNA found in the cerebrospinal fluid (CSF). Also, CSF studies are done to assess the presence of lymphocytes, increased protein level, and glucose level.

2. d.
   The nutritional advice best for a discharged patient taking Coumadin to prevent recurrence of embolic stroke would be to not drink more than two glasses of wine and one mixed drink per week. This is because alcohol causes vasodilation, which leads to increased bleeding.

3. b.
   For the patient about to undergo a lumbar puncture at bedside, the most important part of the nursing preparation is to check the coagulation panel and platelet count. This is to ensure that excessive bleeding does not occur.

4. c.
   Antibiotic therapy is an important aspect of care for the patient with bacterial meningitis because the use of initial antibiotics is based on the most likely causative agent and should be reassessed as soon as CSF lab results return.

5. c.
   For a patient being discharged after an early diagnosis and treatment of Lyme disease, the neurological nurse should stress the importance of finishing all antibiotics.

6. b.
   When caring for a patient with viral meningitis, the nurse should keep the patient in isolation until the patient is afebrile without antipyretics for at least 24 hours, should assess neurological status frequently to detect altered level of consciousness or focal abnormalities, and should implement steps to prevent increased ICP. Maintain head and neck in alignment and start bowel program to prevent stimulating the Valsalva response.

7. a.
   The most URGENT supportive measure needed in preparing the patient for a lumbar puncture is to administer pyretics when fever is present to prevent seizure activity and further complications from the infection.

8. c.
   The most effective way to cool core body temperature during exercise is to drink cool liquids. Other measures include wearing light, loose clothing and maintaining adequate rest and hydration.

9. c.

For a patient with multiple sclerosis who is taking interferon beta-1b, the neurological nurse should explain the goals of therapy and provide support during treatment.

10. d.

For the patient with myasthenia gravis, it is important to educate him/her on a mechanically soft diet as well as on eating small meals. This disease affects the ability to swallow.

11. c.

Treatment for bacterial meningitis is urgent, and the risk of mortality is too great to wait for a definitive bacteriologic diagnosis. Drug selection targets the organisms most likely to be present on clinical grounds and on the known antibiotic sensitivities of those organisms in the region and in the specific institution. These sensitivities vary geographically and evolve over time. Because of the seriousness of the infection, bactericidal antibiotics are preferable. If dexamethasone is included in the treatment regimen, it should be started before—or at least concomitant with—the first dose of antibiotic, as the first phase of bacterial death can intensify the inflammatory response.

12. d.

Unlike bacterial meningitis, viral meningitis cannot be transmitted from person to person via direct contact or airborne secretions. The viruses that cause aseptic meningitis in humans are called arboviruses and are transmitted by mosquitoes. Some of these viruses also cause encephalitis. Serial neurologic examination is important to detect focal neurologic abnormalities as soon as they develop since viral meningitis is often accompanied by encephalitis. Some focal deficits such as dysphagia can be life-threatening. Any deterioration in level of consciousness should also be noted as promptly as possible so that the cause can be addressed, for example, by reversing increased intracranial pressure. Deteriorating level of consciousness is a poor prognostic sign. Hyperthermia in any setting can result in permanent brain damage.

13. a.

Any evidence of a clotting disorder is important because bleeding into the limited spinal subarachnoid space can produce a hematoma that entraps or compresses the cauda equina. The physician will already have assessed the risk of herniation due to increased intracranial pressure with or without a space-occupying lesion. It is advisable to have the patient attend to bathroom needs prior to the lumbar puncture so that he/she doesn't have to sit or stand following the procedure, but this is a lower priority than checking the coagulation studies. No restriction of food or liquid is necessary prior to lumbar puncture. Patient education is a part of preparation for any procedure, but again, the most pressing nursing intervention is to review the coagulation studies.

14. a.

In any patient whose myasthenia gravis is rapidly deteriorating, the most life-threatening development is respiratory failure. This is restrictive rather than obstructive respiratory failure, based on inability of the muscles of respiration to contract sufficiently to move air into the chest. Unlike obstructive failure, restrictive failure is not accompanied by overt respiratory symptoms such as wheezing or gasping, and the patient may not be particularly hypoxic or even feel short of breath until complete respiratory failure is imminent. For this reason, physical examination and arterial blood gases are inadequate measures of pulmonary function, and regular measurement of vital capacity is mandatory. The physician should determine in advance a value at which semi-elective intubation will be instituted in order to avoid a respiratory emergency. It is also important to evaluate other muscle groups, particularly the muscles of swallowing, as aspiration of secretions is also a very serious event. All patients should be carefully monitored for possible adverse events when they start a new medication. A wide range of drugs can worsen myasthenia, and while these are to be avoided, they may sometimes be watchfully given when the potential benefit is judged to outweigh the risk.

15. d.

The key issue is that once a patient loses the ability to swallow or breathe because of ALS, that ability will not return, and intervention is not temporary. Some ALS patients will want to take advantage of every life-saving measure, and some will reject prolonged ventilatory support at the end of life. Many will be ambivalent and need consultation with family members, ethicists, clergy, or other advisors. There may be disagreement among family members. The discussion should be initiated early, respectfully, and supportively.

16. a.

The approximate number of ischemic strokes that occur each year in the U.S. is 700,000.

17. a.

The main cause of an ischemic stroke is a thrombus or clot, which interrupts blood flow.

18. d.

Cardiac sources of embolic stroke include atrial fibrillation, patent foramen ovale, valvular disease, and idiopathic hypertrophy subaortic stenosis.

19. a.

Conditions that can mimic an ischemic stroke are hypoglycemia and unrecognized seizures. Both of these conditions can cause altered consciousness and behavioral changes.

20. d.

The nurse in the emergency department should anticipate a non-contrast brain CT scan for patients with possible acute ischemic stroke.

21. b.

An excessive elevated blood pressure would exclude a patient with acute ischemic stroke from receiving IV tPA.

22. b.

IA thrombolysis can extend the three-hour window of acute-therapy to 12 hours.

23. a.

For the patient with elevated blood pressure who has suffered an acute stroke, the nurse will need to administer Labetalol to control the blood pressure.

24. b.

Prevention of acute complications for patients with ischemic stroke includes intubation and hypertension management. The goal of maintenance of perfusion to the ischemic area involves blood pressure maintenance.

25. d.

A waist circumference of 45 inches increases the patient's stroke risk. The recommended waist circumference for this patient would be less than 35 inches.

26. a.

A blast injury results in a traumatic brain injury where there is damage to the blood-brain barrier as well as to the tiny cerebral blood vessels.

27. d.

The clinical sequelae related to secondary injury sustained with a traumatic brain injury involves possible death; is a complicating injury that often worsens; and can result from a single event, a series of events, or multisystem complications.

28. c.

A severe head injury results in a GCS score of 3 or less, with posturing and airway maintenance issues. The Glasgow Coma Scale (GCS) rates the severity of TBI based on duration of unconsciousness of 21-59 minutes and PTA lasting from 1 to 24 hours.

29. c.

A patient admitted with a sub-acute subdural hematoma will most likely be treated with Burr holes to remove the hematoma, as this removes blood and eliminates intracranial pressure.

30. a.

If a patient starts to have a seizure, the nurse should protect the patient's head and other body parts from injury. Tongue blades and restraints are not indicated.

31. c.

Signs of Cushing response include hypoventilation due to reduced heart rate, increased pulse pressure and blood pressure, and irregular respirations.

32. a.

When a neurologically compromised patient's oxygen level is dropping, the nurse realizes that because of cerebral auto-regulation, cerebral blood vessel dilation will occur.

33. c.

When providing discharge instructions to a patient with a mild brain injury, the neurological nurse should instruct the patient to avoid participating in activities that cause injury because of cumulative effects.

34. a.

A patient with a traumatic brain injury is in need of fluid replacement therapy to maintain a systolic blood pressure of at least 90 mm Hg and should receive normal saline fluids, as the sodium elevates the blood pressure.

35. c.

Nutritional intervention for the patient with a traumatic brain injury includes enteral feedings initiated 72 hours after injury.

36. d.

Coma stimulation for a patient who sustained a traumatic brain injury includes ensuring that only one person at a time is speaking during the exercise.

37. a.

Patients with trigeminal neuralgia should be instructed to eat iced foods and very cold beverages, as this helps with the pain.

38. d.

Broca's (motor) aphasia refers to nonsensical speech that is fluent. Mild to moderate aphasia involves loss of fluency or facility of comprehension without significant limitation on ideas expressed or form of expression. Severe aphasia involves limited communication because there is fragmented expression.

39. c.

A technique used to assess language dominance and memory function before ablative surgery for epilepsy is visual-evoked potential. This is where you sit in front of a screen where alternating checkerboard patterns are displayed. Sensory-evoked potentials involve the use of electrical impulses, which are administered to a leg or an arm. With brainstem auditory-evoked potentials, you hear a series of clicks in the ears.

40. a.
Glasgow Coma Scale (GCS) is a measure of level of consciousness. A GCS score of 13 indicates that a state of confusion is present in an awake, alert patient and is considered a moderate TBI.

41. b.
Therapeutic interventions for increased intracranial pressure (ICP) include administration of mannitol, an osmotic diuretic, administration of corticosteroids, and hyperventilation.

42. d.
Fever, headache, and nuchal rigidity are classic symptoms of meningitis. Other manifestations include malaise, irritability, and vomiting. Meningitis is inflammation of the meninges, caused by bacterial, viral, or fungal pathogens.

43. b.
A condition characterized by the occurrence of small patches of demyelination of the white matter of the optic nerve, brain, and spinal cord is multiple sclerosis (MS). This condition is an acquired, immune-mediated, demyelinating disease of the central nervous system (CNS).

44. d.
The parts of the neuron that receive messages from other cells are called dendrites. Dendrites are short processes with multiple projections that contain cytoplasm, organelles, and neurofibrils. They conduct information to the cell body and receive sensory information from various receptive fields.

45. c.
An electroencephalogram (EEG) is a specific investigation to detect seizures. An EEG confirms the presence of abnormal electrical activity and/or seizures and focality. This non-invasive test is used as a survey of brain rhythms, and a normal recording does not rule out a seizure diagnosis.

46. c.
The most common inhibitory neurotransmitter in the human brain is GABA. GABA is increased in certain neurological disorders. It is a major inhibitory neurotransmitter of mammalian CNS, especially in the cerebellum, spinal cord, and basal ganglia.

47. a.
Donepezil may retard the progress of Alzheimer's disease deterioration. Alzheimer's disease (AD) is characterized by stages and decline in cognitive function. Donepezil (Aricept) is a centrally acting reversible acetylcholinesterase inhibitor. It easily crosses the blood-brain barrier and has an oral bioavailability of 100%.

48. a.

Parkinson's disease is caused by the degeneration of neurons in an area of the brain called the substantia nigra. Research has shown there is a genetic predisposition to PD. There is no single causative agent for PD, but there are several secondary causes.

49. c.

Wernicke's aphasia causes the affected person to be unable to understand or comprehend the language (poor comprehension) with intact repetition (fluent output).

50. d.

Symptoms of Parkinson's disease include tremors of the hands, arms, legs, jaw, and face; stiff limbs; bradykinesia; and impaired balance. Cognition is unaffected with PD.

51. a.

Treatment for epilepsy to eliminate or sharply reduce the frequency of seizures may involve all narrow-spectrum and broad-spectrum antiepileptic drugs, vagus-nerve stimulation, and surgery.

52. d.

Symptoms associated with Guillain-Barré Syndrome include weakening or tingling sensation in the legs, weakness in the arms and upper body, and nearly complete paralysis.

53. b.

Gradually increasing pain and weakness and numbness in the hand or wrist that radiates up the arm suggests carpal tunnel syndrome.

54. c.

Difficulty speaking and understanding speech is called aphasia.

55. d.

A male client has an impairment of cranial nerve II. Specific to this impairment, the nurse should provide a clear path without obstacles for ambulation to ensure patient safety.

56. a.

The most common cause of subarachnoid hemorrhage is aneurysms.

57. a.

Transient ischemic attacks (TIAs) are not permanent. Damage occurs, but the symptoms resolve. With a cerebrovascular accident (CVA), damage and symptoms are permanent if treatment is delayed.

58. b.
The best indicator of changes in neurological function in an alert patient is disorientation.

59. b.
Nursing intervention for the neurological patient should include performing neurological checks.

60. c.
Brief loss of consciousness followed by a lucid period and a secondary loss of consciousness is characteristic of an epidural hemorrhage, which is a form of traumatic brain injury.

61. d.
In a patient with increased intracranial pressure, cerebral perfusion pressure should be maintained at 70mm Hg.

62. b.
The most sensitive indicator of changes in intracranial pressure in unresponsive patients is a change in pupil response.

63. c.
For a patient with a spinal cord injury (SCI) to establish a bladder-retraining program, strategies that may stimulate the patient to void include stroking the patient's inner thigh, pulling on the patient's pubic hair, pouring warm water over the perineum, and tapping the bladder to stimulate the detrusor muscle.

64. b.
For the patient with a spinal cord injury (SCI) who complains about a severe throbbing headache, elevated blood pressure, decreased heart rate, diaphoresis, and flushing, the nurse should check the Foley tubing for kinks or obstruction.

65. b.
The patient with multiple sclerosis is easily fatigued. In this situation, the appropriate nursing diagnosis would be activity intolerance due to generalized weakness.

66. b.
For the patient with an acute hemorrhagic stroke, alteplase is not indicated. This drug is used primarily for patients who have a myocardial infarction.

67. a.
The patient who had a stroke and needs to be fed should be positioned in the Fowler's or semi-Fowler's position.

68. b.

The patient with bacterial meningitis who complains of a severe headache with photophobia and who has an oral temperature of 102.6° F should be given an infusion of ceftriaxone (Rocephin) 2,000 mg IV.

69. d.

The information obtained during a patient's chart review and assessment that would be most concerning is that the patient wishes to renew his driver's license.

70. d.

For a patient with a recurrent glioblastoma who is receiving dexamethasone (Decadron) 4 mg IV every six hours to relieve symptoms of right arm weakness and headache, it would be concerning if he/she experienced a significant weight gain.

71. b.

A CT scan of the head would be indicated, since his/her symptoms include lethargy, confusion, incontinence, and sleepiness.

72. a.

When caring for the intensive care unit (ICU) patient with meningococcal meningitis, the student should wear a gown and mask.

73. f.

When creating a teaching plan for a patient with newly diagnosed migraine headaches, the key items that should be included are: avoiding foods with tyramine, avoiding certain medications (Tagamet, nitroglycerin, and Nifedipine), using abortive therapy, instructing about medication side effects, and providing complementary relaxation therapies.

74. b.

A client admitted to an emergency department who is "postictal upon transfer" has recently experienced a seizure and is drowsy and confused.

75. c.

To confirm the presence of an acoustic neuroma, that patient should have a magnetic resonance imaging (MRI) test.

76. c.

A depressed injury is one in which the scalp and skull remain intact, but the underlying tissue is damaged.

77. d.

An excessive accumulation of cerebrospinal fluid (CSF) is known as hydrocephalus. This occurs as a result of a clinical syndrome and is not permanent.

78. c.
A chronic disturbance of the nervous system characterized by recurrent seizures that are the result of abnormal electrical activity of the brain is known as epilepsy.

79. d.
A contusion is where the brain tissue is bruised, blood from the broken vessels accumulates, and edema develops, causing increased intracranial pressure (ICP).

80. d.
When admitting a patient who has a tumor of the right frontal lobe, the nurse would expect to find speech difficulties. Aphasia and apraxia occur secondary to various prefrontal cortex lesions.

81. a.
For the patient with a basal skull fracture, clear drainage from the patient's nose could indicate leakage of cerebrospinal fluid (CSF). The questionable order would be insertion of a nasogastric tube.

82. b.
A patient with a neck fracture at the C5 level who has neurogenic shock will have hypotension, bradycardia, and warm extremities. This is secondary to autonomic dysfunction that occurs with injuries at and below the level of T6.

83. b.
A patient with a head injury who opens his eyes to verbal stimulation, who curses when stimulated, and who does not respond to a verbal command to move, but attempts to remove the painful stimulus would have a Glasgow Coma Scale score of 11.

84. b.
In the patient with the presence of Cushing's triad, the nurse would expect to find a decreased pulse, irregular respirations, and an increased pulse pressure.

85. a.
A patient has intracranial pressure (ICP) monitoring with an intraventricular catheter. A priority nursing intervention for the patient is aseptic technique to prevent infection, but other interventions include monitoring for changes in vital signs and neurological status.

86. d.
Metabolic and nutritional needs of the patient with increased ICP are best met with a balanced, essential diet that the patient can tolerate.

87. c.
Cranial nerve three (CN III) originating in the midbrain is assessed by the nurse for an early indication of pressure on the brainstem by testing pupillary reaction to light.

88. a.
For a patient with risk for ineffective cerebral tissue perfusion related to cerebral edema, an appropriate nursing intervention is to avoid positioning with neck and hip flexion.

89. c.
Because posturing can increase ICP, the nurse should perform range of motion (ROM) exercises less frequently.

90. d.
The presence of an arterial epidural hematoma should be suspected in the patient who experiences unconsciousness at the time of a head injury, with a period of consciousness followed by decreased level of consciousness.

91. d.
A patient with a depressed parietal fracture with a subdural hematoma should be taken to surgery for a craniotomy for evacuation of blood and decompression of the cranium.

92. a.
The nurse's first priority in management of the patient once a patent airway is confirmed would be to maintain cervical spine precautions.

93. b.
Frontal lobe tumors present many symptoms and challenges for the patient. These lesions cause difficulty with memory, mood swings, decreased concentration, and trouble with multitasking.

94. b.
Classic symptoms of bacterial meningitis include high fever, nuchal rigidity, and severe headache. Insidious non-specific illness starts with fever, malaise, irritability, and vomiting. This progresses over two to four days, and when rapidly fulminating illness develops within 24 hours, it can produce a poor outcome.

95. b.
The best way to position a patient with increased ICP is to elevate the head of the bed to 30°. Head elevation can decrease ICP related to increased cerebrospinal fluid and/or venous drainage from the intracranial space as a result of gravity.

96. c.
The nurse on the clinical unit should assess first the patient with meningitis who is suddenly agitated and reporting a headache of 10 on a 0 to 10 pain scale. This indicates the possibility of increased intracranial pressure and other complications.

97. d.
Domain 5: Safety includes crisis management and risk management.

98. b.

The nurse should encourage the patient with multiple sclerosis to rest in an air-conditioned room. Multiple sclerosis is an acquired, immune-mediated, demyelinating disease of the central nervous system (CNS). One of the symptoms of MS is increased temperature sensitivity, so the room should be kept cool for these patients.

99. a.

A patient with Guillain-Barré Syndrome may have paralysis affecting the respiratory muscles that requires mechanical ventilation, but all patients experience some recovery. Only 15-25% experience residual weakness.

100. a.

The nurse working on a surgical floor must logroll a male client following a laminectomy. During the recovery phase, the nurse should increase the patient's activity level gradually, as tolerated. Also, the nurse should monitor neurological function and assess for complications.

101. b.

Before a CT scan, the nurse should determine whether the patient is allergic to iodine, contrast dyes, or shellfish, as allergies to these would contraindicate the test.

102. b.

When assessing deep tendon reflexes, the nurse should make sure to support the joint where the tendon is being tested.

103. d.

For a client admitted in a disoriented and restless state after sustaining a concussion during a car accident, the priority nursing diagnosis would be risk for injury.

104. b.

A female client with amyotrophic lateral sclerosis (ALS) should have a diagnosis of "powerlessness," due to the nature of the disease.

105. c.

A client may be ineligible for a magnetic resonance imaging (MRI) diagnostic procedure based on his/her history of a prosthetic valve replacement.

106. d.

Before a lumbar puncture is performed, the nurse should place the patient in the side-lying position with the legs pulled up and the head bent down onto the chest.

107. b.
For a patient with increased intracranial pressure, the nurse should place the patient with his/her head turned to the side.

108. d.
For a male client with a spinal cord injury who is prone to experiencing automatic dysreflexia, and to minimize the risk of recurrence, the nurse should limit bladder catheterization to once every 12 hours.

109. b.
For the patient with complete right-sided hemiparesis, the nurse should understand that he/she is weak on the right side of the body including the face and tongue.

110. a.
For the client with a brain attack (stroke) who has residual dysphagia, when a diet order is initiated, the nurse should avoid giving him/her thin liquids.

111. d.
After a brain attack (stroke), the nurse should encourage the consistent use of adaptive equipment when dressing.

112. c.
For the patient who has had a brain attack (stroke) and aphasia, the nurse should speak slowly, allow the patient plenty of time to respond, and look directly at the patient during attempts at speech.

113. c.
For a patient with myasthenic crisis, the nurse would assess whether he/she has precipitating factors such as omitting doses of medication.

114. a.
Bell's palsy cause is unknown, but is possibly related to ischemia, a viral infection, or an autoimmune problem.

115. d.
The patient has probably experienced a transient ischemic attack (TIA), which is a sign of progressive cerebral vascular disease. A TIA is a temporary focal loss of neurologic function caused by ischemia of an area of the brain; usually, this lasts only about three hours. TIAs may be due to microemboli from heart disease or carotid or cerebral thrombi and are a warning of progressive disease. Evaluation is necessary to determine the cause of the neurologic deficit and to provide prophylactic treatment, if possible.

116. c.
Involves removing an atherosclerotic plaque in the carotid artery to prevent an impending stroke. An endarterectomy is a removal of an atherosclerotic plaque; plaque in the carotid artery may impair circulation enough to cause a stroke. A carotid endarterectomy is performed to prevent a cerebrovascular accident (CVA), as are most other surgical procedures. An extracranial-intracranial bypass involves cranial surgery to bypass a sclerotic intracranial artery. Percutaneous transluminal angioplasty uses a balloon to compress stenotic areas in the carotid and vertebrobasilar arteries and often includes inserting a stent to hold open the artery.

117. d.
Maintenance of respiratory function with a patent airway and oxygen administration. The first priority in acute management of the patient with a stroke is preservation of life. Because the patient with a stroke may be unconscious or have a reduced gag reflex, it is most important to maintain a patent airway and provide oxygen if respiratory effort is impaired. IV fluid replacement, treatment with osmotic diuretics, and perhaps hypothermia may be used for further treatment.

118. c.
Daily low-dose aspirin. The administration of antiplatelet agents such as aspirin, dipyridamole (Persantine), and ticlopidine (Ticlid) reduces the incidence of stroke in those at risk. Anticoagulants are also used for prevention of embolic strokes, but they increase the risk for hemorrhage. Diuretics are not indicated for stroke prevention other than for their role in controlling blood pressure, and antilipemic agents have been found to significantly effect stroke prevention. The calcium channel blocker nimodipine is used in subarachnoid hemorrhage patients to decrease the effects of vasospasm and minimize tissue damage.

119. b.
Surgical clipping of the aneurysm. Surgical management with clipping of an aneurysm to decrease re-bleeding and vasospasm is an option for a stroke caused by rupture of a cerebral aneurysm. Placement of coils into the lumens of the aneurysm by interventional radiologists is increasing in popularity. Hyperventilation therapy would increase vasodilation and the potential for hemorrhage. Thrombolytic therapy would be absolutely contraindicated, and if a vessel is patent, osmotic diuretics may leak into tissue, pulling fluid out of the vessel and increasing edema.

120. c.
Alteplase is used for acute ischemic stroke in adults because it improves recovery and reduces the incidence of disability. Treatment with this drug is initiated within three hours after onset of the stroke symptoms and after exclusion of intracranial hemorrhage by cranial CT or other diagnostic imaging methods.

Exclusive Trivium Test Tips

Here at Trivium Test Prep, we strive to offer you the exemplary test tools that help you pass your exam the first time. This book includes an overview of important concepts, example questions throughout the text, and practice test questions. But we know that learning how to successfully take a test can be just as important as learning the content being tested. In addition to excelling on the CNRN, we want to give you the solutions you need to be successful every time you take a test. Our study strategies, preparation pointers, and test tips will help you succeed as you take the CNRN and any test in the future!

Study Strategies

1. Spread out your studying. By taking the time to study a little bit every day, you strengthen your understanding of the testing material, so it's easier to recall that information on the day of the test. Our study guides make this easy by breaking up the concepts into sections with example practice questions, so you can test your knowledge as you read.
2. Create a study calendar. The sections of our book make it easy to review and practice with example questions on a schedule. Decide to read a specific number of pages or complete a number of practice questions every day. Breaking up all of the information in this way can make studying less overwhelming and more manageable.
3. Set measurable goals and motivational rewards. Follow your study calendar and reward yourself for completing reading, example questions, and practice problems and tests. You could take yourself out after a productive week of studying or watch a favorite show after reading a chapter. Treating yourself to rewards is a great way to stay motivated.
4. Use your current knowledge to understand new, unfamiliar concepts. When you learn something new, think about how it relates to something you know really well. Making connections between new ideas and your existing understanding can simplify the learning process and make the new information easier to remember.
5. Make learning interesting! If one aspect of a topic is interesting to you, it can make an entire concept easier to remember. Stay engaged and think about how concepts covered on the exam can affect the things you're interested in. The sidebars throughout the text offer additional information that could make ideas easier to recall.
6. Find a study environment that works for you. For some people, absolute silence in a library results in the most effective study session, while others need the background noise of a coffee shop to fuel productive studying. There are many websites that generate white noise and recreate the sounds of different environments for studying. Figure out what distracts you and what engages you and plan accordingly.
7. Take practice tests in an environment that reflects the exam setting. While it's important to be as comfortable as possible when you study, practicing taking the test exactly as you'll take it on test day will make you more prepared for the actual exam. If your test starts on a Saturday morning, take your practice test on a Saturday morning. If you have access, try to find an empty classroom that has desks like the desks at testing center. The more closely you can mimic the testing center, the more prepared you'll feel on test day.
8. Study hard for the test in the days before the exam, but take it easy the night before and do something relaxing rather than studying and cramming. This will help decrease anxiety, allow you to get a better night's sleep, and be more mentally fresh during the big exam. Watch a light-hearted movie, read a favorite book, or take a walk, for example.

Preparation Pointers

1. Preparation is key! Don't wait until the day of your exam to gather your pencils, calculator, identification materials, or admission tickets. Check the requirements of the exam as soon as possible. Some tests require materials that may take more time to obtain, such as a passport-style photo, so be sure that you have plenty of time to collect everything. The night before the exam, lay out everything you'll need, so it's all ready to go on test day! We recommend at least two forms of ID, your admission ticket or confirmation, pencils, a high protein, compact snack, bottled water, and any necessary medications. Some testing centers will require you to put all of your supplies in a clear plastic bag. If you're prepared, you will be less stressed the morning of, and less likely to forget anything important.
2. If you're taking a pencil-and-paper exam, test your erasers on paper. Some erasers leave big, dark stains on paper instead of rubbing out pencil marks. Make sure your erasers work for you and the pencils you plan to use.
3. Make sure you give yourself your usual amount of sleep, preferably at least 7 – 8 hours. You may find you need even more sleep. Pay attention to how much you sleep in the days before the exam, and how many hours it takes for you to feel refreshed. This will allow you to be as sharp as possible during the test and make fewer simple mistakes.
4. Make sure to make transportation arrangements ahead of time, and have a backup plan in case your ride falls through. You don't want to be stressing about how you're going to get to the testing center the morning of the exam.
5. Many testing locations keep their air conditioners on high. You want to remember to bring a sweater or jacket in case the test center is too cold, as you never know how hot or cold the testing location could be. Remember, while you can always adjust for heat by removing layers, if you're cold, you're cold.

Test Tips

1. Go with your gut when choosing an answer. Statistically, the answer that comes to mind first is often the right one. This is assuming you studied the material, of course, which we hope you have done if you've read through one of our books!
2. For true or false questions: if you genuinely don't know the answer, mark it true. In most tests, there are typically more true answers than false answers.
3. For multiple-choice questions, read ALL the answer choices before marking an answer, even if you think you know the answer when you come across it. You may find your original "right" answer isn't necessarily the best option.
4. Look for key words: in multiple choice exams, particularly those that require you to read through a text, the questions typically contain key words. These key words can help the test taker choose the correct answer or confuse you if you don't recognize them. Common keywords are: *most*, *during*, *after*, *initially*, and *first*. Be sure you identify them before you read the available answers. Identifying the key words makes a huge difference in your chances of passing the test.
5. Narrow answers down by using the process of elimination: after you understand the question, read each answer. If you don't know the answer right away, use the process of elimination to narrow down the answer choices. It is easy to identify at least one answer that isn't correct. Continue to narrow down the choices before choosing the answer you believe best fits the question. By following this process, you increase your chances of selecting the correct answer.
6. Don't worry if others finish before or after you. Go at your own pace, and focus on the test in front of you.

7. Relax. With our help, we know you'll be ready to conquer the CNRN. You've studied and worked hard!

Keep in mind that every individual takes tests differently, so strategies that might work for you may not work for someone else. You know yourself best and are the best person to determine which of these tips and strategies will benefit your studying and test taking. Best of luck as you study, test, and work toward your future!